A Singular View

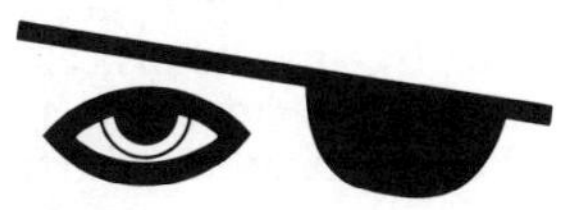

A Singular View

The Art of Seeing With One Eye

Frank B. Brady

U.K. Edition
Edited by Ron Hearnden

Edgemore

Canadian Cataloguing in Publication Data

Brady, Frank B.
A singular view: The art of seeing with one eye.

The Art of Seeing With One Eye.

U.K. ed.

ISBN 0-9695534-0-4

1 Vision, Monocular. 2. Visually handicapped - Rehabilitation. 3. Vision disorders. I. Hearnden Ron.
II. Title

RE95.B73 1992 362.4'1 C92-093549-4

Previously Published in Canada by Edgemore Enterprises Inc. Toronto Ont.
ISBN 0-9695534-9-4

Previously Published in the USA by Frank B. Brady, Annapolis, Maryland, 21403
ISBN 0-9614639-1-0

Previously Published in the USA by Medical Economics Books, Oradell N.J., 07649

Printed and bound in Great Britain by The Bath Press.

Published by
Edgemore Enterprises Inc.
P.O. Box 127
260 Adelaide St. East Post Office
Toronto, Ontario.
M5A 1N1

U.K. Distribution By
Lavis Marketing
73 Lime Walk
Headington
Oxford
0X3 7AD

Contents

Foreword

By John W. McTigue, M.D., F.A.C.S.

When Frank Brady told me that he was toying with the idea of writing a "a sort of manual for the newly one-eyed," my response was instant and positive. "That is a book that should be written," I told him, "and you're the one to do it."

Frank Brady can speak with the authority of a person who was forced to adjust to the loss of an eye in the very prime of his life. Because of his extensive background in air navigation and in developing ways of landing planes under poor visibility conditions, he was quickly able to understand the problems created by the destruction of so complex an instrument as the human eye. And he tackled those problems with an uncanny problem-solving ability.

In no time he was driving a car, flying a plane, plunging into sports with skill and enthusiasm, working as effectively as ever at his highly technical job, and courting the girl who is now his wife.

Mr. Brady made this remarkable adaptation almost entirely without benefit of guidance, because — no such guidance was available. There are schools and training centres and many books available for persons with practically any type of handicap you can name, including those totally without sight. Yet, as far as I know, there has never been anything even vaguely resembling this sort of "manual for the newly one-eyed."

A child born with only one good eye, or who loses vision in one eye at a very early age, never faces the adjustment problems that plagued Frank Brady after his accident. A one-eyed child adapts to his limited vision as naturally as the normal child does to binocular sight. Unconsciously and unselfconsciously, he learns a whole battery of compensating techniques that the child with two good eyes never needs to know — techniques for gauging depth and distance and for enlarging his restricted field of vision.

The fact that such a child can go on to lead a completely normal life — without any sense of being handicapped — should, I suppose, give hope and reassurance to the person who loses an eye after growing up. Indeed, a return to normal living is equally possible for him. Yet I'm afraid this crumb of comfort isn't enough to help him through the often difficult period of adapting to his new situation.

Each year, an estimated 10,000 Britons enter the world of the one-eyed — most of them without advance notice. The loss of an eye is usually sudden and traumatic — by injury or accident — and may plunge its victim into an immediate depression. Reminding him that little Alfie, who was *born* with only one eye, has just graduated at the top of his class isn't going to cheer up an adult victim very much.

Nor will it help him cope with the immediate problems and vexations he'll encounter in everyday activities — all the errors of visual judgment that will make him feel anxious, clumsy, foolish. The ophthalmologist may tell him he's going to "carry on as before," but rarely does a busy physician have time to sit down with such a patient and explain precisely *how* to "carry on as before." Even if he did, he could never have that special understanding of the patient's problems that can come only from experiencing them.

This book fills that gap admirably. The author starts out with a vivid though understated description of his accident and his feelings when he learned that his damaged eye would have to be removed. He recounts the tribulations and failures in his early efforts to get back to his old way of life with his new restriction. He tells us how he mastered each of his problems in turn.

There follows a remarkably condensed and simplified basic course on how the human eyes function, with particular reference to depth perception and visual field. We learn exactly what a person with monocular vision has lost and what's necessary for an intelligent adaptation to living with one good eye.

I particularly like the chapters that follow — the nuts-and-bolts of the book. Here Mr. Brady explains his techniques for shaking someone's hand without missing, for stepping off a kerb without stumbling, for guiding a car through a narrow lane or a thread through a needle's eye. He makes the obstacles and pitfalls appear much less challenging as he leads us on through the world of gadgetry — glasses, magnifiers, rangefinders, offset gunsights, and other ingenious devices to improve performance of specific tasks.

Frank Brady's observations on lighting, a field that cries out for more research, may prove to be a pioneering contribution.

The next chapter — the one he discussed most with me — tells the newly one-eyed how to care for and make the most of the precious eye that's left. This is followed by some useful information on licensing requirements for car drivers and plane pilots.

A chapter new with this edition is For Parents Only. In it, Mr. Brady gets parents off to a good start in helping their newly one-eyed children adjust to monocularity — psychologically as well as physically.

The book ends with a reminder that loss of an eye late in life didn't cramp the style or detract from the achievements of some world-famous people working in a variety of fields.

While this manual is addressed primarily to the newly one-eyed, I hope that it will reach the much larger audience it deserves. It should make almost equally good reading for those who have long ago adapted to what Mr. Brady refers to, not as a handicap, but as "this inconvenience," or "this damned nuisance."

I think this book will also interest anyone who is

curious about the workings of one of nature's most fabulous creations — the human eye. And it will certainly captivate every person who enjoys reading about man's amazing capacity for adaptation.

Preface

A man's eyes are his closest bond to his environment, and any threat to his vision is certain to produce massive anxieties. Even the loss of *one* eye can be a matter of enormous concern to an active individual in love with living. Will he ever, he wonders, be able to work again, to drive, to fly, to hunt, to win a mate, even to manage to cross a road.

I went through all these anxieties when I lost my own good right eye, but I suppose I tended to feel that my reactions were exceptional. It really wasn't until friends began to call on me to help reassure others who had recently lost an eye that I began to understand how deep the psychological trauma inflicted by loss of an eye.

These sessions also brought home to me the fact that there is very little guidance for the newly one-eyed during the long, awkward, and sometimes dangerous period of adaptation. The experiences I went through while getting used to monocular vision prompted me to develop techniques for newcomers — practical suggestions that could help them over the kerbs and staircases and other stumbling blocks on the road to normality.

Publisher's Notes

Frank B. Brady is a resident of Annapolis, Maryland. A Professional Engineer, registered in the District of Columbia, he has a broad background in aviation and electronics and recently retired as Executive Director of The Institute of Navigation, a Washington based technical and scientific society. He is a recognized authority in the field of aircraft all-weather landing, electronic and visual aids to navigation and does independent consulting in these fields.

Mr. Brady was able to draw both on his technical education and on his professional experience in coping with the problems that come from loss of vision in one eye. This book is a by-product of his success in solving these problems. He is the author or co-author of some three dozen technical papers and articles plus a large number of reports in various fields of aviation technology. He has served as an expert witness in court cases involving eye loss.

John W. McTigue, M.D., F.A.C.S., who wrote the foreword and served as medical consultant of the U.S. edition of this book, is chief of the department of ophthalmology at the Washington Medical Center in the District of Columbia. He is past president of the District of Columbia Medical Society's section on ophthalmology; past president of the Prevention of Blindness Society, Washington, D.C.; associate medical director of the International Eye Foundation, Washington, D.C., and a member of the board of directors of the Eye Bank Association of America. His primary professional interests are diseases and surgery involving the cornea. He is the author or co-author of more than 20 professional papers.

Ron Hearnden was born and still lives in Toronto where he is President of Edgemore Enterprises Inc. and also is sales manager of one of Canada's largest book manufacturers. He has spent most of his working life in the paper and printing industries.

Ron lost his right eye at age of 40 as a result of a fall while skiing "one of, if not the, smallest hills" in Ontario. He resumed his business career immediately after recovering from the surgery that removed his right eye, with a new position that required travel across North America. The lessons learned from this book helped Ron to recognize potential problems and how to adapt to them.

Acknowledgments

One of the most pleasant surprises connected with the preparation of this book has been the enthusiastic response to almost any request for assistance. I couldn't possibly acknowledge all the help I've received from individuals and organizations, but I do want to mention a few that have been especially generous with their resources. These include:

The American Medical Association's Committee on Medical Aspects of Automotive Safety.

The Federal Aviation Administration, Office of Aviation Medicine.

The American Association of Motor Vehicle Administrators.

The American Optometric Association.

The Guild of Prescription Opticians of America.

American Society of Ocularists

Mr. Joseph Murphy, editor and publisher of *Airline Executive* magazine, who helped me find a publisher.

My acknowledgments wouldn't be complete without a word of appreciation for Dr. Wendell Hughes, the eminent New York ophthalmologist who brought patience and delicate skill to the performance of five operations over a two-year period that succeeded in rebuilding my battered features.

And finally, a heartfelt thank-you to Dr. John W. McTigue, the distinguished ophthalmologist in Washington, D.C., without whose encouragement, prodding, and generous assistance this book might never have got beyond the procrastination stage.

Editor's Notes

My thanks to Linda McKnight of MGA, a great literary agent and a good friend who guided me through the acquisition process and gave invaluable help in developing this book.

Jeremy Brown of Newcastle Publishing, who was kind enough to edit the editor for the most nominal of fees, my profound thanks.

This book would not be complete without acknowledging the contribution made by Mrs. Kay Davies of DVLC, Graham Phillips of Big Type, Ashley and Janice Scott at Bath University, Ms. Marjorie Allan of the British Standards Institute, Jack McCabe of The Bath Press, and Dr. R. A. Pearson of the Civil Aviation Authority.

This edition of A SINGULAR VIEW probably would not have been produced without the support and assistance of Mr. J. J-p. Atwill, House Governor and the medical staff of Moorfields Eye Hospital. This world renowned facility provided much of the information regarding eye care.

I especially want to acknowledge the help and

researching done for this book by my daughter Lisa Hearnden. Her insistence in her father learning the rules of the road in Britain was the motivation for this edition. It was worth all those collect transatlantic telephone calls.

In Canada, we had the help of Mrs. H. Marshall, Information Officer at the British Consulate, Ian Paterson, vice president of Imperial Optical Company, and Dr. Silvio Finkelstein of the International Civil Aviation Organization.

The technical advice of George R. Metcalfe, proof reader extraordinaire and Gerard Williams for his cover and text design ensured that we had a good looking book.

I would be remiss not to acknowledge Guy Lefevbre and Gagne Printing for their support and encouragement, I am sure that they thought that I never would finish this project. Thanks for the use of the computer.

FINALLY, I have to thank Frank Brady for writing the book. It made a great difference to me in being able to cope with a dramatic change in lifestyle. I learned that it is the little things like pouring drinks that will do you in. Not the major problems that you would expect. Frank has been an inspiration to me and thousands of others who had to learn to adapt to "A SINGULAR VIEW".

Ron Hearnden

1 Unhappy Landing

I have no memory of being hit. I recall only a dazed awareness that something was wrong, very wrong...that Charles Macatee was swinging our plane into position for a landing...asking the tower for runway lights...calling for an ambulance to meet the plane.

Then Tom Wright, the third man aboard, was helping me out of the cockpit, where I had been flying co-pilot, and onto a couch so that he could take my place and assist in the landing.

Interminable minutes later (less than three, actually), I was being lifted into the ambulance. Exactly seven minutes after the accident, I was getting skilled emergency treatment in an Air Force hospital.

Our plan, a research DC-3, had been on the last leg of a flight from Chicago via Washington that April evening.

We'd been skimming over Long Island after sunset

and were preparing to land at Grumman Field, when the craft was struck. Captain Macatee had no idea what had hit us until after landing, when he found a five-pound mallard duck in the cockpit.

The big bird, one of a migrating pair that had collided with us, had crashed through the windshield and struck me full in the face, bouncing my head against the aluminum bulkhead behind me. A large dent in the heavy metal testified to the force of that blow. Later, when I had a chance to examine it, I realized that the bulkhead had actually kept my neck from snapping.

In my work in aviation safety, I had taken a keen interest in a procedure designed to test the resistance of cockpit windshields to just such bird strikes. The method was to fire a newly-killed chicken, encased in a paper bag, from a pneumatic cannon at various types of windshield mock-ups.

The technique is still in use today, except that the chickens are now fired at velocities as high as 700 miles an hour. Thanks to such testing, the modern cockpit windshield is an inch-thick marvel of strength, with heated laminations to prevent its becoming brittle at high-attitude temperatures.

By a wry twist of fate, stronger windscreens had been ordered installed on all DC-3s. Ours arrived shortly after the accident.

2 Awkward Takeoff

It was several days before the doctors decided I was strong enough to hear the bad news: My right eye had been damaged beyond repair. It would have to be removed without further delay, they told me, in order to prevent a sympathetic reaction from developing in the good remaining eye.

The verdict didn't really surprise me, even though the damaged eye had been kept under wraps all this time. And there was really no point in brooding about it. I began instead to develop an overwhelming curiosity about the future. Would my world be changed when viewed through a single eye? Would my activities be restricted? Would I ever drive a car again? Fly a plane? Play golf or even just cross a road with a reasonable expectation of reaching the other side alive?

In the course of my life, I'd met quite a few people

who had lost the vision of one eye. Now I spent long hours in my hospital bed anxiously trying to recall all the details I'd learned about them so I could apply this knowledge to my own circumstances.

There was Bob, for instance, who wore a patch on one eye and delighted in driving his car at 90 miles an hour on winding rural roads, scattering alarm throughout the countryside. I had no desire to duplicate Bob's madness, but at least it was heartening to think that the loss of half his vision had restrained him no more than the laws of the land.

On the other hand, I knew that Bob had lost his eye at a very early age, and I wondered if this might not be the key to his amazing adaptation. Could I, already past 30, hope to win back enough of my old skills — to say nothing of acquiring some necessary new skills — to continue the life I'd been leading?

My thoughts turned, this time more hopefully, to another acquaintance — one who had lost an eye when he was already a grown man. Cliff, a co-worker in an engineering lab, won the respect of all of us for his impeccable craftsmanship. He had often discussed with me some of the techniques he used to gauge distances and manipulate instruments — techniques that were presently to serve me well.

Then there was the great Wiley Post, one of my boyhood heroes. With only the relatively crude instruments of the period, Post had twice circled the globe by air with only one good eye to guide him. Pondering his long solo flights and his many landings under the most difficult conditions helped to convince me that having undergone the loss of one eye need not necessarily handicap me for the rest of my life.

So my mind drove on, searching out reasons for optimism and answers to doubts. But the trip wasn't all upbeat. A hospital environment has a way of magnifying fears and misgivings to unrealistic proportions, especially at night, and there were times when I felt agonisingly sure that neither my personal nor my professional life would ever be the same again.

On the day set for my discharge from the hospital, a pleasant young man came into my room and introduced himself as Dr. Drake.

"How're you doing?" he asked.

"I'm just fine," I answered truthfully. The prospect of being able to get back into action at long last had buoyed my spirits.

Dr. Drake sat down and began what seemed to be a very casual, amiable, and innocent conversation. But little by little, his questions became more penetrating, dwelling especially on my general outlook about life. He wanted to know whether it had changed in any way since the accident.

It was only near the end of the interview that I began to realize I was on the receiving end of a very skillful psychiatric examination. Dr. Drake's purpose, obviously, was to find out whether the loss of an eye and the battering of the whole right half of my face had thrown me into a depression.

The effect of the interview, however, was to raise my mood almost to the point of elation. I began to feel a bit like the boy in the story who asked the doctor, after surgery on his hands, "Do you think I'll be able to play the piano now?"

"Definitely," said the doctor.

"Wow!" screamed the boy. "That's great! I could never do *that* before."

Apparently, I emerged from the interview with passing marks, for when Dr. Drake rose to go he wished me good-bye and good luck.

I reached to grasp his outstretched hand — and missed by a mile!

3 Jolts of Reality

It didn't take me too long to master the art of handshaking, but the real world that was waiting to wake me up from my hospital daydreams had many more rude jolts in store for me.

Outside the hospital, I hailed a cab and stepped off the pavement as it approached. Underestimating the height of the kerb, I jolted forward and nearly ended up under the taxi's wheels.

At a party in my honour, I volunteered to mix a martini for a thirsty young woman. I mixed it perfectly. Then, when she held up her glass to receive it, I poured it on the floor.

My "grand entrance" at another party became a spectacle. I descended the stairs, raised my hands in greeting the guests, stepped into the living room, and fell forward in amazement. The last step had disguised itself as part of the living room floor.

My first try at table tennis was a disaster that stirred my friends to a pitying quietness.

It seemed everybody in the world had suddenly decided to move in on my right (sightless) side, and I was in a constant state of collision with them. A restaurant waitress serving hot soup on my right came up just as my hands were describing the size of a fish I'd once caught. I caught the plate this time, and a painful burn that lingered on my right arm for several days — evidence of a newborn clumsiness.

For some time, I was to live in a world of clumsiness and embarrassments, much of which I could have been spared if only someone had given me the explanations and helpful tips that appear in the following chapters.

It was perhaps with justifiable trepidation that at the urging of friends I got behind the wheel of a car two days after leaving the hospital. I tried to cling to the left lane, but I found it hard to judge my distance from the parked cars and the double-parked cars. And terrors seemed to spill in from all directions at the crossroads — but particularly from the right.

I had to swivel my head in much wider arcs, much faster and much more frequently that I ever had before, and I needed a heightened alertness to cope with each new danger. I was pathetically grateful for the "co-pilot" on my left during the first nightmarish ride through town.

Out on the open motorway, however, things went

more smoothly, and some of my former ease at the wheel returned. I did become aware, however, of a tendency to overrun the car ahead. But I quickly learned to lag a little farther than usual behind vehicles and soon began to understand why my old friend Bob had no qualms about going 90 miles an hour once his path was clear of traffic.

It was while driving at slow speeds, threading my way between other cars on the city streets, or backing into a parking space that I experienced the most serious difficulty in judging distances. Nevertheless, I ended that first drive with the certainty that this was one activity I wouldn't have to give up, for at no time had I felt that I was driving in an unsafe manner. Any loss of visual perception was more than offset by the enforced — and often excruciating — increase in alertness.

4 Flying High

That same super-alertness sustained me as I tested myself in a variety of skills for which I had a well-established know-how — but also a recently acquired uneasiness about my do-how. For it was back in my boyhood that I had begun acquiring the assortment of knacks and knowledges that later guided my choice of a career.

At 16, I was a glider buff, obtaining my pilot's license in a craft that school chums and I had built and taught ourselves to fly. Soon after that, I became fascinated by amateur radio, building and operating amateur stations. And as I grew up, I was drawn almost painlessly into the field of radio engineering. My old interest in flying, however, led me to aviation electronics, where I found a new specialty — the development of instrument approach and landing systems.

World War II created a demand for men with this type of background, and as a young civilian engineer I was soon in charge of a sizable instrument landing programme for the Allied Forces in Europe. After the war, I joined the civil aviation industry to help the airlines adapt to peacetime use the new air traffic control and instrument landing systems that had proved so successful. It was in this capacity that I was directing a flight research programme on the night of the accident.

Though my main interest had always been my work, I don't think I was backward in social or outdoor activities. Swimming and sailing were my favourite sports, augmented by a bit of tennis and golf. Now each of these old activities presented new challenges as I cautiously experimented and, problem by problem, worked out ways of coping.

Shortly after the accident, I was back at my job and having no difficulty filling it. The flight research programme had been dropped, so I was no longer required to fly. I flew anyway — partly to find out how I'd do at it and partly because it's in my blood. In many ways, I found it easier than driving, and I had no trouble with making the distance judgments that are required for landing and other manoeuvres.

Even today, with increased air traffic making it imperative for a pilot to keep a sharp lookout in the sky, I find that the super-alertness I've trained into myself since the accident easily compensated for the loss of side vision. In fact, I would go so far as to say that there is a *net gain* in safety.

Perhaps my most demanding post-accident project

was the building of a ship model to exacting standards. It's true that threading all those tiny deadeyes, setting up the rigging at a scale of one-eighth inch to the foot, and doing all the other fine detailed work wasn't easy; the point is that it could be done — and done with no loss of quality in the workmanship.

All in all, my adaptation was well along at the end of a year. By the end of two years, I was totally at ease in all normal activities, even though I was, for cosmetic reasons, still undergoing plastic surgery. Some jobs took a little extra time and effort, and many situations called for the hyper-awareness I've already mentioned. But if I sometimes regarded my new condition as a damned nuisance, I never considered it a handicap — in my career, in my hobbies, or in my personal life.

It was toward the end of this rehabilitation period that, through a chance meeting, my personal life took a highly affirmative turn and the success of my adaptation was proved by the fact that for months I made weekly trips from Washington up through Maryland and Pennsylvania, driving seven hours at a stretch — and mostly at night — to woo the future Mrs. Brady.

5 How About You?

So much for my story. Now what about yours? If you're reading this book, the chances are that you've just lost, or are in the process of losing, the full use of one eye. In the months ahead — those months that now occupy all your thoughts — will you fare as well as I did? Better? Worse? Let's take a look at some of the factors that may help or hinder you on the road back.

Every person is right-eyed or left-eyed, just as he is right-handed or left-handed, depending on which half of the brain is dominant. The right hand, foot, and eye are controlled by the left hemisphere of the brain, which in most people is dominant. Obviously, the loss of your right hand, if that's the favoured one, would call for a far longer and more difficult readjustment than loss of the left; it would entail a massive re-education of the brain.

To a lesser extent, the same holds true of the eyes. If

your brain is accustomed to receiving messages and making decisions on the basis of information received from your right eye, and that's the one you lose, the road back is going to be a bit more arduous for you. In my own case, it was the right, or favoured, eye that was removed, so it was a minus factor for me.

While eye dominance is perhaps the single most important factor of the prognosis, there are many others that play a part. One of these is acuity of vision. If the surviving eye has good vision (as in my case), it can more readily take over the functions of its lost mate, even though that mate may have been the favoured one. But if the surviving eye has poor vision and is also the secondary eye, then it's going to take more time and effort to adjust.

Age, of course, is another important factor (the younger you are, the better). So is the gradualness or the suddenness of the loss. If the deterioration of one eye goes on over a long period of time, the good eye has a chance to accustom itself slowly to the increased work load and make an orderly transition. That is, provided the deterioration doesn't cause troublesome symptoms that could retard your adaptation.

Then, of course, much depends on how far you want or need to carry your adaptation. Some occupations (such as mine) and some hobbies (such as mine) call for more accurate depth perception than is normally required. Achieving this requires a longer and more determined effort than average, too.

Of extreme importance is each individual's psychological reaction to the loss of an eye. And here the difference between any two people can be striking, ranging all the way from "What's the use of living?" to "I hardly notice the difference."

One night, while I was still in the early stages of my own recovery, I got an urgent call from a friend asking whether I would please talk with his 18-year-old nephew, who had recently lost an eye as the result of a car accident. Fred, he said, had come home from the hospital in such a severe depression that his family was greatly concerned about what he might do and didn't know how to help him. I readily agreed to visit. I thought that it might also be helpful to me.

It turned out that Fred and I had a lot more in common than the loss of an eye. During our conversation, I learned that he was a glider enthusiast, and immediately I was able to talk his language. As soon as we got on to that subject, he told me the cause of his despair, which, very simply, was that he was certain he'd never again be able to fly a glider.

I was able to assure him from my own experience that he was completely mistaken. I told him about some of the tricks I'd learned to compensate for my loss of vision while flying. At last he was convinced, and his mood quickly changed from one of self-destruction to eagerness to get on with his recovery.

But not all psychological reactions to the loss of an eye are so simple. I've known victims who took it as a punishment for God knows what unspeakable sins they'd committed in their imaginations. Others feel they must *over*compensate for the loss by learning to do *more* than they could when they had normal vision. The miseries and frustrations that can come from such reactions sometimes call for prolonged psychiatric help.

On the other hand, some people of great character and determination actually become even greater successes by overcompensating — like Sammy Davis Jr. When this great entertainer had the top rung practically in his grasp in 1954, a car crash damaged his left eye beyond repair. While recuperating, he vowed: "When I come back, there can be no 'He's almost as good as he ever was.' I've got to be better."

And within four months he was back, this time right at the top of his profession. Nothing sick about that!

6 Seeing in 3-D

If you've enjoyed fairly normal vision since birth, it may never have occurred to you that a great deal of what we call "seeing" is really a learned skill. We tend to take it for granted that any creature born with eyes can "see." But show a dog a photograph of his beloved master, and he'll display no sign of recognition whatever. It takes an educated brain to be cable to see in the shapes and variations of colour on a piece of paper the likeness of a human being.

I once witnessed the reaction of a small boy who was watching his father's plane take off from a private airfield. As the small plane soared away into the blue, the child began to scream.

"Daddy will be back soon" his mother reassured him. But that wasn't what was bothering the boy.

"Look!" he screamed even louder, pointed to the tiny speck in the sky, "Daddy's getting *small!*"

The youngster was only confirming what scientific studies have found — that the gift of sight doesn't necessarily endow a person with "perception," or the ability to grasp the meaning of what he sees. People who had been blind from birth, and then suddenly have eyesight conferred on them by surgery or some other technique, have a whole new language to learn. It takes them some time, for instance, before they can interpret perspective in a picture — just as it must have taken the little boy some time to learn to relate small size to distance.

In the same way, partial loss of the vision you've learned and have used all your life entails a completely new learning experience. But there's a tendency among people who've always had normal vision to make the transition from two eyes to one by letting nature take its course. This unorganized approach will eventually get you there, but you can speed it up and smooth it out significantly by doing a bit of homework. The first thing you need to understand is the nature of the change that has taken place. What is it, exactly, that you have lost? And what is it that you have left?

The human eye is certainly one of nature's most amazing creations. Just as man stands at the top of the evolutionary ladder, vision is the most highly developed of the sense. Each eyeball is in reality a superbly crafted sub-subminiature camera. When both these cameras are in good working order, their owner need only raise his eyelids to obtain a continuous view of the world in glorious 3-D living colour.

Most owners use their cameras for fixed viewing about 90 percent of the time. During the remaining 10 per cent, the cameras swivel back and forth, up and down, in a series of rapid movements, scanning various parts of the surrounding scene at the rate of two or three "takes" per second.

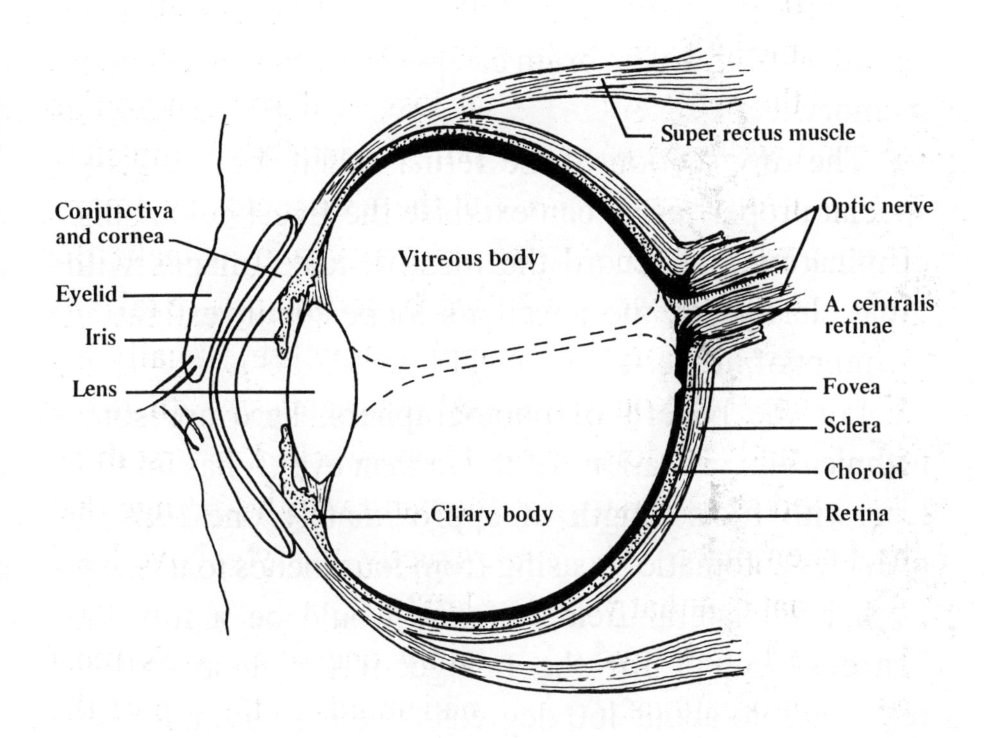

Sectional diagram of the human eye.

Any part of the big scene that commands the owner's attention, whether it be the top of a mountain or the eye of a needle, first enters the eye through the cornea. This tough, transparent outer shell of the eyeball serves two purposes: (1) it protects the delicate mechanisms from injury, and (2) its front surface bends the rays of light passing through it to form the image on the retina. The lens, by changing shape, provides the change in focus required for viewing near and far objects.

The retina, of course, corresponds to the sensitive film of the movie camera. And just as the images can be stored on film, so the brain can preserve them back in its memory.

The tiny section of the retina called the fovea has special properties. It can exercise the finest colour discrimination and record the most delicate images with great clarity. It's the jeweller's loupe for investigating the point of interest.

For the benefit of photographers, here are some technical specifications of the human eye: It has an f3.5 lens with focal length of approximately one inch. It provides automatic focusing from four inches to infinity. Each eye's lateral field of view would be a full 180 degrees, except for the bridge of the nose, which restricts it to about 160 degrees. The iris automatically adjusts the pupil opening by a factor of 16 to one to accommodate extremely wide variations in light levels. The eye sees in such detail that it can resolve about 10 lines pairs per millimetre at normal reading distance.

It's true that a hawk can see better than a man at great distances, and that a cat can see better in the dark. But for man's all-around viewing purposes, there's certainly nothing better than a human eye.

Except, perhaps, two of them.

7 What's Changed?

What happens, physiologically, when you lose one of those two optical marvels with which you've been viewing the world? You know, as soon as you step back out into that world, that *something* has happened, because it's suddenly been transformed into a china cupboard. Your adaptation to this new and uncomfortable environment can be speeded by an elementary understanding of what's taken place *inside* of you.

Three things have happened:

• Your horizontal field of vision has narrowed.

• Your depth perception has been impaired.

• Your whole visual system, including brain and motor functions, is in disarray and needs reprogramming so the two can be able to work together in integrated fashion.

Other, minor, effects will be touched on later. But first let's consider these three important ones.

Field of vision

You've literally lost by a nose here. As we remarked in the last chapter, each eye has a lens capable of taking in everything on the horizon within 180 degrees, or a full

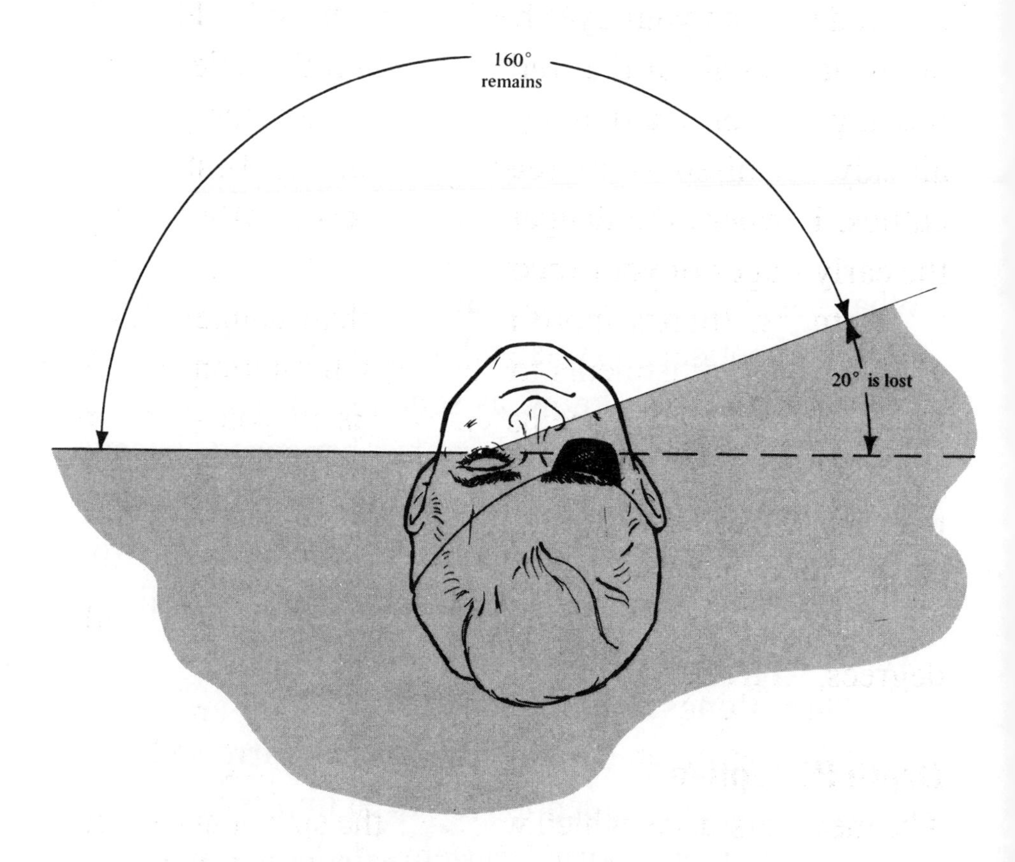

Depending on nose size, the horitzontal field for one eye will encompass up to 160°, compared with a 180° field for normal, two-eyed vision.

half circle. But that bony prominence in the middle of your face cuts off anywhere from 20 to 40 degrees of that view, depending, naturally, on its size and shape.

This was no problem, of course, so long as you had a good eye on the other side of your nose. Each eye was then able to stand sentinel over that area its mate couldn't cover.

With one eye gone, the total field of view once covered by both your eyes has been reduced by 10 to 20 per cent, and all of that reduction is on the side of the missing or nonfunctioning eye. That side, as you've already surmised from reading about my first difficulties, is where the danger lurks — especially during the early stages of your recovery.

Actually, there's more nuisance than danger, once you've made adjustments to your new limitation. If the loss of lateral vision seems enormous to you — as it usually does at first — keep in mind that it's really less than many people with two good eyes inflict on themselves voluntarily by wearing heavy-rimmed glasses.

Your *vertical* field of vision, which total around 130 degrees, won't be affected.

Depth Perception

The mechanisms by which we judge the size of an object and its distance from us are much more complex than most people realize. In part, this is because psychological factors often have an important influence on such judgments. If, for example, you lay a coin and a metal

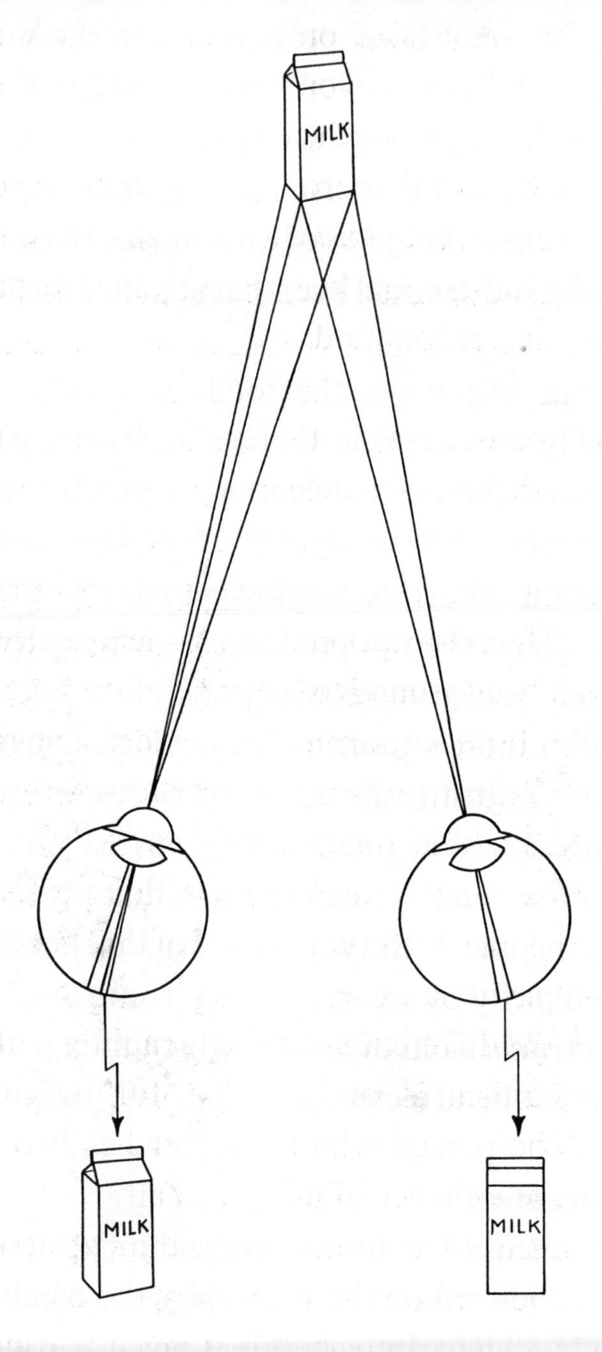

Retinal disparity — each eye seeing a slightly different image — helps the brain compute size and distance of objects. One-eyed people have lost this mechanism.

washer the same size on a table and ask an underprivileged child to tell you which is larger, the odds are heavy that he'll choose the coin.

However, depth perception also involves several pretty sophisticated *physiological* operations. In medical terminology these are known as retinal disparity, convergence, and accommodation.

RETINAL DISPARITY is the most obvious and widely known of these mechanisms. It depends on an object being viewed with two eyes separated by several inches so that each eye is looking at the same target from a slightly different location at the same moment. One eye sees a little way around to the right of the object, and the other eye a little way around to the left. The result: Two slightly different images are produced on the two retinas. Before these images are merged into one clear picture, the brain examines the differences and uses them to make a swift computation of the object's size and how far away it is.

Since the differences diminish rapidly with distance, this mechanism is of little use for judging remote objects. The person who no longer has two good eyes doesn't have a chance of using it at all.

CONVERGENCE has to do with the merging of the two images produced on the retinas by the mechanism just described. The effort by the eyes to bring the two images into exact correspondence produces a strain, or torsion, on each eye, and the experienced brain knows how to translate this into a measure of distance. The closer the object, the greater (and more measurable) the torsion. And if you've ever looked cross-eyed at a pencil held vertically in front of your nose, you've experienced this strain at its extreme.

Like the mechanism of retinal disparity, convergence is useful only at relatively small distances (25 feet or less), and only people with binocular vision have it.

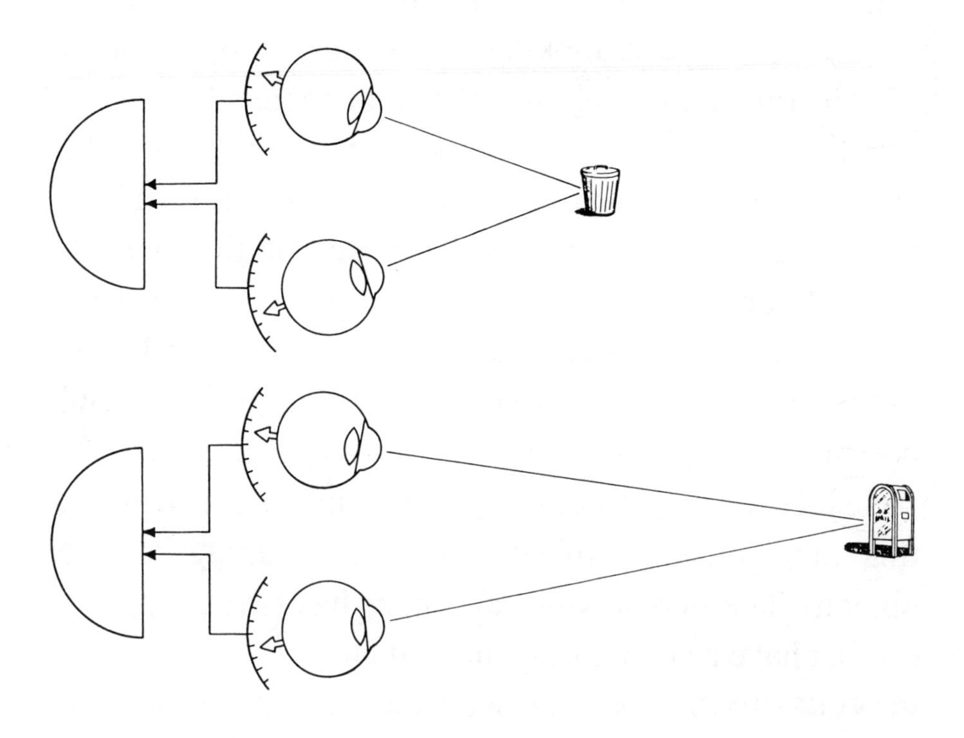

Convergence — the rangefinder mechanism — allows the brain to compute distances based on the different angles from which each eye sees an object.

ACCOMMODATION is a term for the automatic adjustment each eye makes to bring an object into focus (as distinct from adjustment, already described, which is then made to merge the two images). This is accomplished by changing the curvature of the lens, and the muscular

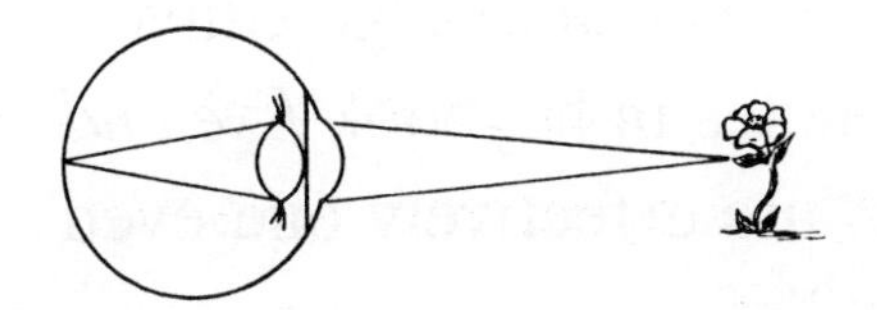

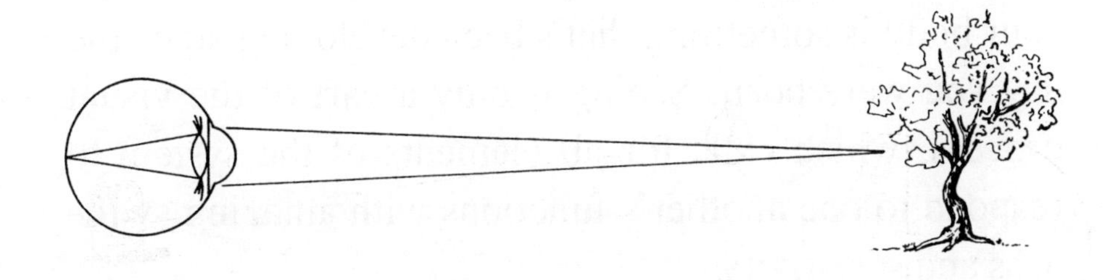

Accommodation — the change in curvature of the lens to bring objects into focus — is immediately interpreted by the brain as a measure of distance.

effort required to do so is immediately registered on the brain as a measure of distance.

Accommodation is only effective for judging distances up to about six feet; thus it's likely to be the least useful of the three mechanisms. But it's the only one left to you when you've lost an eye, so cultivate it for what it's worth. You'll soon learn, however, that there's greater gain in developing new techniques to compensate for the loss of retinal disparity and convergence.

Bear in mind, too, that compensation is necessary only up to a point. R. L. Gregory of Cambridge University's psychology department notes in his book *Eye and Brain* that *all* sighted persons "are effectively one-eyed for distances great than 20 feet."

The Visual System

The relationship between your eyes, your brain, and your body is something that's been developing since the day you were born. Seeing is only a part of the visual process, which calls for all elements of the system to respond to one another's functions with amazing swiftness and sensitivity.

Even as you read this book, your brain, receiving a signal from your eye, consults its own vast memory bank in order to make a judgment about it. It then sends out its commands via the nervous system to activate the body's motor systems. "Turn the page," says your brain, and your fingers obey.

What happens when your brain receives an impaired

or different visual message — one for which it has no precedent in its memory bank? To understand how the visual system can be disorganized, let's picture a batsman who is about to swing at a bowled ball.

He's trained himself to judge the speed and path of the ball by any or all of the three physiological depth-perception processes we've just talked about. A fourth factor he sometimes brings into his computations is the angle at which the ball is approaching the wicket. The angle changes as the ball nears, and the brain has the ability to convert the information on the degree of the change into a prediction as to where and when the ball will cross the crease. Having digested all available information, the brain at the proper instant sends out a command to the proper muscles to swing the bat. Then, if all goes well, the ball and bat connect solidly at exactly the right juncture in time and place.

But suppose we ask this batsman to close one eye and repeat the performance. Only one of the three build-in depth perception techniques — accommodation — is now available to him. And as we know, it won't do him any good until the ball is practically on top of him. So he's forced to rely very heavily on information derived from the angle of the ball's approach.

But his techniques for observing the angle have not really been sharpened (as they would be if this had always been his sole criterion). His brain's filc on the subject of cricket angles is still sparse. In short, it's a good bet that he's going to miss the ball.

Even if he has been a highly skilled cricketer, a significant part of his skill will be lost in the transition from dual to single vision. If instead of just closing one eye experimentally, our batsman had actually lost the use of that eye permanently, he'd have to develop a whole new set of skills. He'd have to supply his brain with a whole new complex of signals and experiences to store for future reference. And if he was a professional, he may never regain the level of skill he had before.

Most amateurs in the same situation, however, should certainly be able to get back enough skill to enjoy the game. And many may find, as I so often did, that a slight loss in ability can be more than made up by an increase in effort and attention. In fact, in many less critical sports than cricket, there's no reason why the loss of an eye should be any problem at all.

8 Getting Back to 3-D

Have you ever seen a photographer cover one eye to study a scene before he films it? What he's trying to do, of course, is to view the picture in two dimensions, the way his one-eyed camera will view it.

And that's an example of the way you'd view the world from now on, if you took the loss of one eye lying down — or sitting still. Sitting in your room with your head motionless, you no longer see a little to the right and a little to the left of every object to give it roundness and depth. Your eyes no longer strain to bring two slightly different images into correspondence on your retinas. Thus deprived of the two most important physiological means of depth perception — retinal disparity and convergence — what you see is a rather flattened-out scene, much like an ordinary photograph.

Now tilt your head back so that your eye moves up a couple of inches. Something happens. Everything in the room shifts position a little. The edge of the chair in front of you seems to go down a trifle, the television set behind it to come up a trifle, so that you see a bit more of the TV

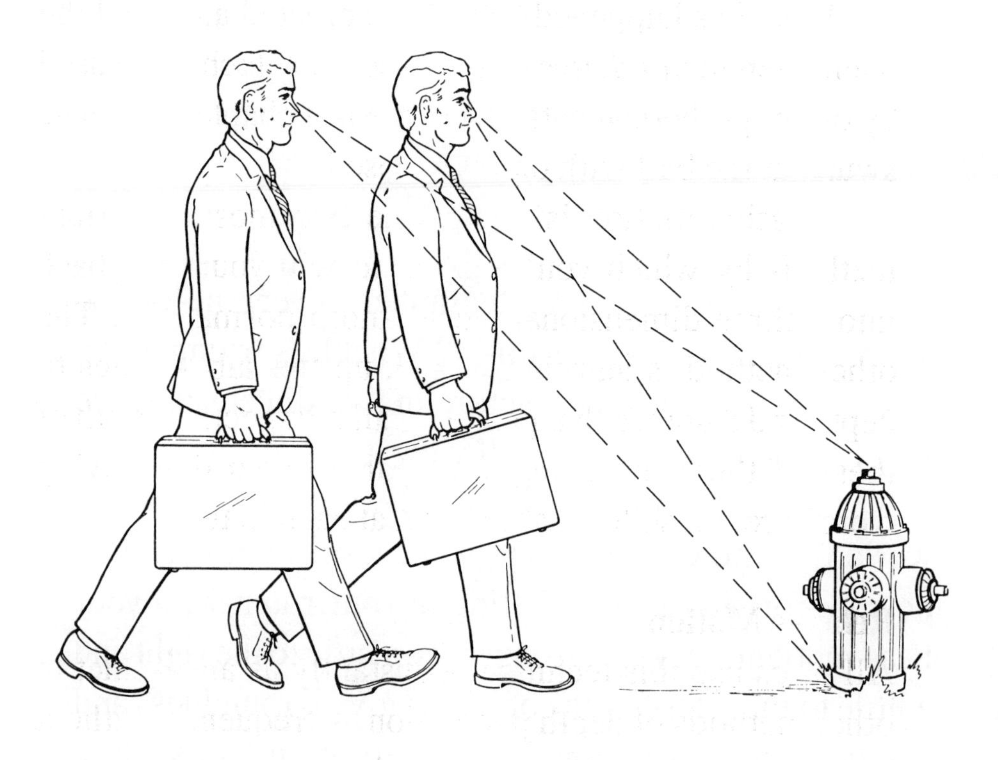

Relative motion — the varying angles and the apparent change in size of objects as you move toward or away from them — will be your primary technique in regaining depth perception.

screen. Your brain at once translates the degree of shift into an estimate of the distance between the TV set and the chair, and for an instant you are able to see your surroundings in three dimensions again.

Perhaps your brain's estimate was off by a hair or a hand. No matter. With practice, you're going to become quite accurate at this kind of estimating. In fact, it's going to become a way of life with you.

What has happened? You have created and used the phenomenon of *relative motion*, the same technique used by our hypothetical batsman in the last chapter, when he swung at the ball with one eye closed.

Relative motion is one of the two most important methods by which you're going to win your way back into a three-dimensional world and a normal life. The other method is learning to pick up the subtle clues to depth and distance that painters call perspective. Both of these methods are going to be part of your daily living from here on, so let's take a look at each in turn.

Relative Motion

All of us use this technique constantly as an adjunct to other methods of depth perception — frequently without being aware that we're doing so. For the one-eyed person, a grasp of the principles involved is an important shortcut to full adaptation.

One final reference to our batting friend out there on the pitch. He was able to use the principle of relative motion because he was standing *to one side* of the wicket at which the ball was aimed. Consequently, the ball sped toward him at an angle, which kept changing as it approached. Without this angle, his brain would have had little to work on in computing his swing.

Now let's leave the cricket pitch and move to a tennis court. Here we'll ask you to imagine yourself behind the net with a hard ball coming directly toward you. As it

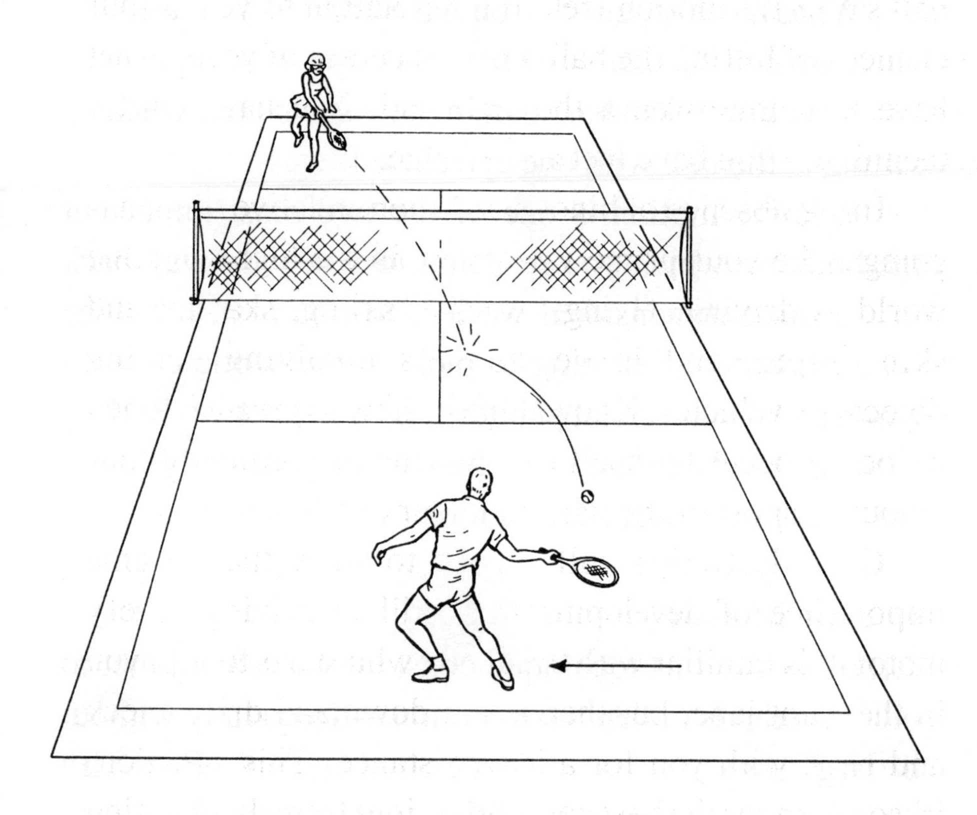

Correct tennis position is suited to the needs of the one-eyed player. It's always to the side, out of the path of the ball. A quick shift of position, when the ball is coming head on, creates the angle a one-eyed player needs to judge where the ball is going.

approaches, there's no change in the angle of its path — just an apparent increase in its size, which is not enough information for your brain to accurately compute your swing at it.

What do you do to remedy this situation? Shift your position. With one quick movement, place yourself off to the side, which is the proper tennis position. This creates the angle of approach your brain needs to compute the ball's relative motion (relative in relation to you). Your chances of hitting the ball with the centre of your racket have now improved a thousandfold. You have used a technique. You have met a challenge.

In the absence of binocular vision, relative motion is going to be your prime visual tool in the highly mobile world of driving, flying, boating, skiing, skating, and skin diving, and in occupations involving moving objects or vehicles. Knowledge of how to create it when it doesn't occur by itself can hasten your return to your favourite sport or the wheel of your car.

One illustration will suffice to show the extreme importance of developing this skill in driving. Every motorist is familiar with the driver who starts to pass you in the right lane, but then slows down and drives neck and neck with you for a long distance. This situation, irksome under the best conditions, is extremely irritating to the one-eyed driver. Even though both cars are travelling at high speed, the relative motion between them is zero. This means that the one-eyed driver has very little in the way of clues to the distance between the two cars.

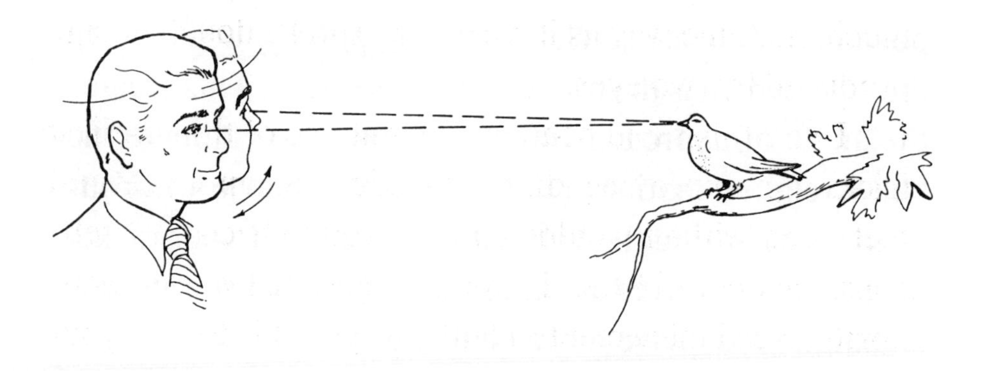

A quick side movement of your head will give you slightly different views of an object. This simulation of binocular vision creates a sense of perspective, especially at close range.

What's the prescription here? Change speed. Go a little faster or a little slower than he does. The result is relative motion and a much improved ability to judge the distance between the two cars. It's often that simple to sharpen your depth perception and manoeuvre yourself out of a dangerous situation.

When viewing a stationary object at short range, one very effective way to produce something akin to relative motion is to move your head quickly to one side. This not only creates a slight shift of the object against its background (as did the up-and-down head movement described earlier in this chapter), it also enables you to have two slightly different views of the same object in such rapid sequence that the brain can interpret them in much the same way as it would interpret a double image produced by two eyes.

I find this rapid head movement one of the handiest tricks for improving distance judgment up to several feet. And while I wouldn't advise you to become a self-conscious swivel head, I would suggest that you use your normal head movements as fully as possible to give your world a third dimension.

Perspective

We turn to the world of art for other important methods of improving depth perception. In their endless quest for ways of depicting a three-dimensional world on a two-dimensional canvas, painters long ago came up with several techniques that can be equally useful to you in reverse — that is, in trying to convert your relatively flattened out world back into 3-D. All these techniques can be lumped under the general term "perspective."

Let's stand at a window — preferably one commanding a view — and ask the great Leonard da Vinci to join us. Leonardo's descriptions of how he used light, colour, and shadow to gain realism and depth in his immortal paintings have much to teach us. With the old master's help, we notice three important facts about the scene outside our window:

• Objects in the foreground take up more of the window's space than objects of the same size in the distance. Automobiles, which are fairly standardized in size, are a good gauge of this. Leonardo calls this phenomenon "diminishing perspective."

• Colours are bolder and brighter in the foreground. In the distance, they become softer and muted. By the same token, shadows of nearby objects are sharper and darker. The artist calls this "colour perspective."

• Finally, objects in the distance tend to blur, while those in the foreground are more clearly defined — the "vanishing perspective."

These observations are as precious to the one-eyed person as they are to the painter, for each of them can be translated into improved depth perception. It's a process you can hasten by consciously applying your attention to it — and as a fringe benefit you'll find the world a far more fascinating place to view.

While the rules of perspective are simple, their application to a given scene is sometimes tricky. An automobile right in front of you takes up much more of your field of vision than it does two blocks away. But since you already know its *size*, you can use its *apparent* size to estimate its distance from you.

If you know the *distance* of an object from you — for instance, if you see a round object bobbing in the water at the end of a pier whose length is familiar to you — it's not hard to estimate the round object's size. But if neither distance nor size is known to you, you'll have to look for other clues.

A principle used extensively in flying and boating can be extremely useful in such situations. Suppose, while you're sailing a boat on a straight course, you see another boat (of unknown size at an unknown distance) moving on a path that will eventually cross your. Seasoned pilots warn their students to "beware of a flyspeck on the windshield that doesn't move but just keeps getting bigger!"

The thing to watch for is the angle of the other boat's path in relation to you. If the angle changes, and continues to change, the boat will pass clear. Beware if there's no change in angle.

This navigation technique, which was developed for normally sighted people, is even more useful to the person with only one eye.

9 Pitfalls and Booby Traps

If your experience is anything like mine when you return to your everyday environment after the loss of an eye, you'll feel suddenly beset with pitfalls and booby traps of all descriptions and on every side. Identifying each one is half the battle; developing a technique to come is the other half.

Nearly all the troubles you're likely to get into are traceable to two factors: loss of depth perception and reduction in field of vision caused by the existence of your nose. In the previous chapter, we discussed some tricks for regaining depth perception in given situations. But the only way to cope with the cutoff on the sightless side of your nose is to develop the habit of looking around — *before* you leap. This means that you will go through life using your neck more than your did.

What follows is a rundown of some specific situations that can bring you bumps, jolts, embarrassments, bruises, and even more serious griefs if you aren't ready for them — along with a specific antidote for each.

Shaking Hands

Of all my early experiences in adaptation to one-eyed vision, none caused more chagrin than reaching out to grasp a friendly hand and closing my fingers on thin air — and none is more easily avoided.

The point to remember is that you don't have to know exactly how far you are from the object you're reaching for in order to connect with it. It's not so much a question of distance judgment as it is of alignment.

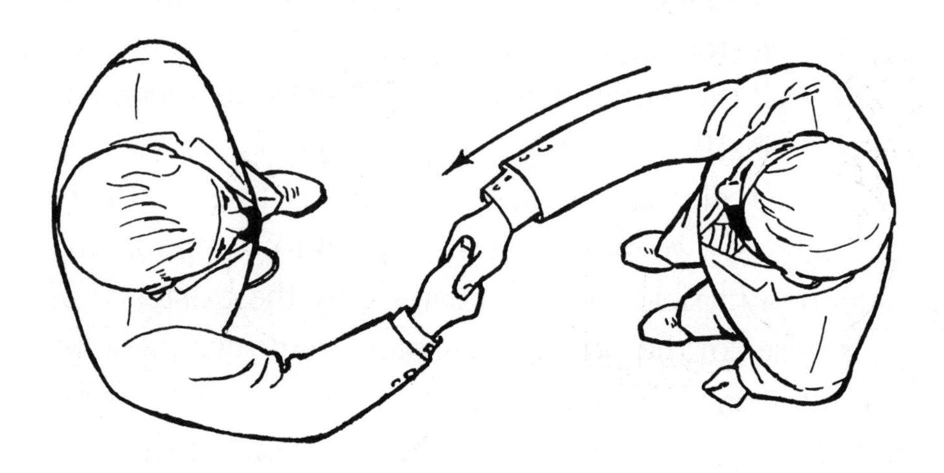

You should have little or no trouble in making contact with an object if you first remember to line up with it and then simply keep on extending your arm and hand until you touch it.

To perform this simple act with complete confidence, simply move your hand in a direct line toward the hand you wish to shake — and keep on moving until you connect. The technique, of course, is equally useful in reaching for a doorknob, a hanger in a wardrobe, a book in a bookcase, or a glass of water on a table.

Pouring

The distance judgment required to pour accurately from one container (e.g., a martini jug) into another (e.g., a

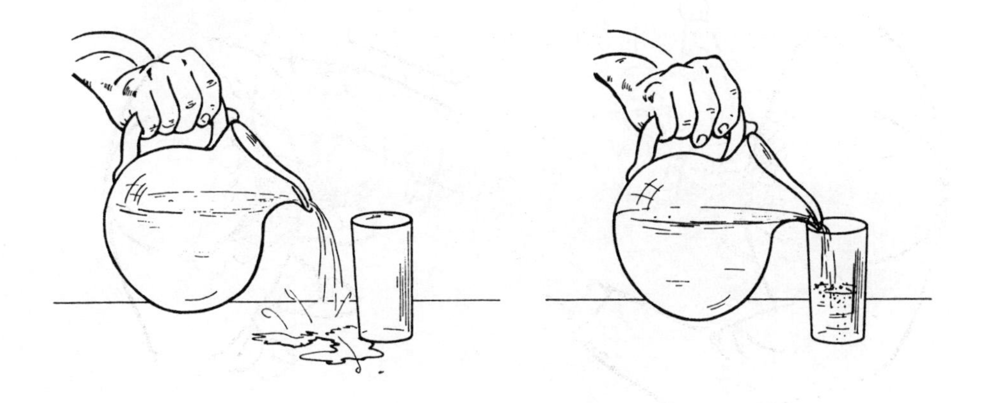

Experience will bring distance judgment necessary to pour from one container to another without missing. Until then, pour with the upper container touching the rim of the lower.

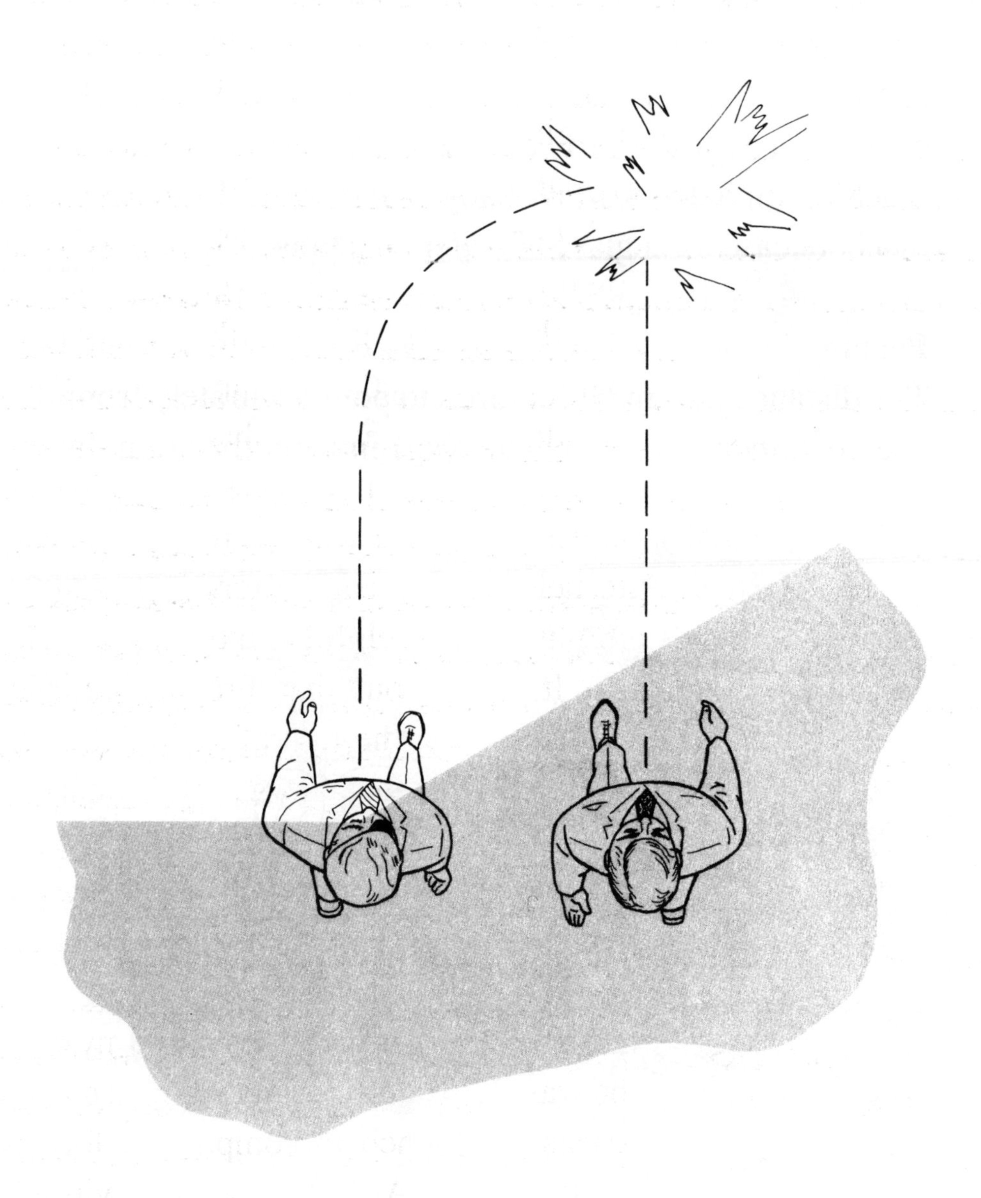

Whether you're out walking, driving, skiing, flying, or skating, always take a good look around before you make any sudden turns.

cocktail glass) comes with a little experience. But until then, it's surprisingly easy to miss your aim completely.

If you want to avoid the kind of spillage I was constantly apologising for in my early days out of the hospital, here's a childishly simple yet sure technique: Place the spout or lip of the upper container right down over the rim of the lower one so that they actually touch, then pour with abandon — you can't miss! By resting the neck of your sugar spoon on the edge of your coffee cup in the same manner, you can make sure that *all* the sugar gets into the coffee.

The Collision Course

"I'm forever bumping into people," is one of the most common complaints of the newly one-eyed. You'll find these collisions nearly always occur when you make an abrupt turn toward the side on which your vision is partly cut off, that is, into the blind spot you checked only a moment ago and found empty.

Moral: "A moment ago" simply isn't enough to take care of the danger. Check that blind spot the very instant you're ready to make your turn. That way no Sneaky Pete will take you by surprise.

The habit of checking probably won't "set" until you've had quite a few bumps. But cultivate it carefully in all situations that involve change of direction — particularly where safety is involved, as in swimming ,skiing, riding, skating, or boating, and most especially in driving and flying. Before you change lanes on the motorway, take a *very* good look around to make sure a mini or similar vehicle hasn't crept up and is lurking just outside your field of vision.

Dining

I've often noticed that a left-handed person will choose a seat at the table where he won't tangle with a right-handed person when they start to eat. In the same manner — when it doesn't violate protocol or carefully worked out seating arrangements — I choose a seat that I hope will favour my good eye.

I find that if I'm required to keep up a conversation with a partner on my right, which happens to be the side of my visual cutoff, the excessive amount of head twisting involved can be not only tiring but annoying. An engaging dinner partner may be worth the extra effort, but if you can make prior arrangements to favour your good side, everyone will be happier.

But remember that the choice of the best seat for conversation doesn't always eliminate other dining dangers. If the meal is being served by a waiter — especially a skilled, *unobtrusive* one - he may be at your sightless side the very moment you least expect him. A few bad experiences with well-trained waiters taught me to take a deliberate look at the right before making any unusual gestures in that direction.

You should be luckier in your situation, now that you've been forewarned.

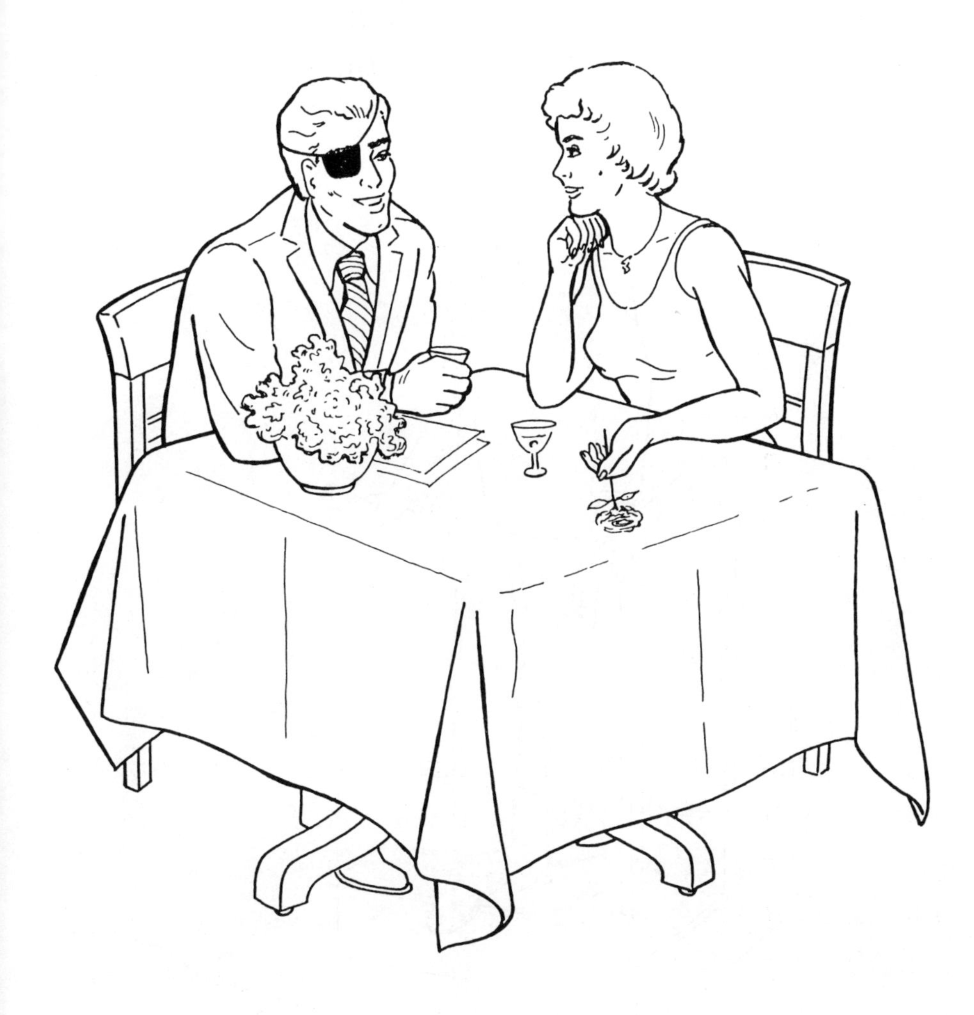

When dining, remember to choose a place at the table that favours your good eye, and watch out for waiters serving on your sightless side.

Staircases

Whether you're going up or down, *watch that last step!* Viewed with one eye, it may blend right into the floor above or below it — especially if it has the same carpeting or finishing treatment and if the light is dim. In

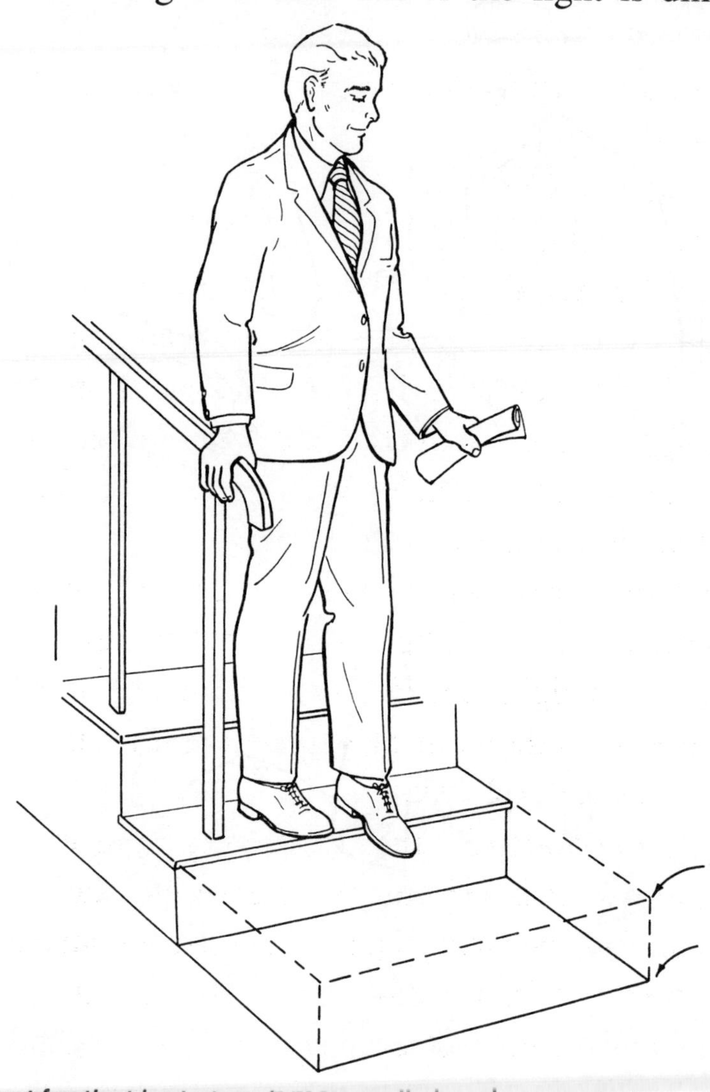

Look out for that last step. It may really be above or below where you think it is, especially when tread and floor coverings are the same.

either direction, it's all too easy to assume that you've taken the last step and start walking away, only (jolt!) to discover that there was one more.

This illusion can be particularly dangerous for the elderly. But anyone who has lost his binocular vision should take that last step gingerly — feeling ahead with his toe and keeping one hand on the handrail.

Kerbs

A close relative to that last step of the staircase, the kerb can be even more treacherous. As you'll quickly discover, kerbs show surprisingly nasty variations in height from one street corner to the next. There are no handrails to hold onto, and a single misjudgment could easily jolt you into the middle of traffic.

After this dire warning, I'm sure you'll immediately start practicing the simple trick I've discovered for estimating the height of a kerb without benefit of binocular vision. It uses the same principle of relative motion that we've already explored.

As you approach the street, keep your eye on the edge of the kerb so you can observe its relative movement against the background of the street's surface. The higher the kerb, the faster will this relative motion appear and the more street paving will it bring into view. Your brain will have no trouble at all computing these factors, along with your walking speed, and will send you a message telling you just how deep a step to take when you hit the street.

With a little practice (and I suggest that you do your *initial* practicing in a safe place) the technique will become so much a part of your adaptation that you won't even have to think about it. It'll serve you equally well wherever you have to judge the distance between two horizontal surfaces. Once you've learned it, you need have no qualms about accepting an invitation to go mountain climbing or go spelunking.

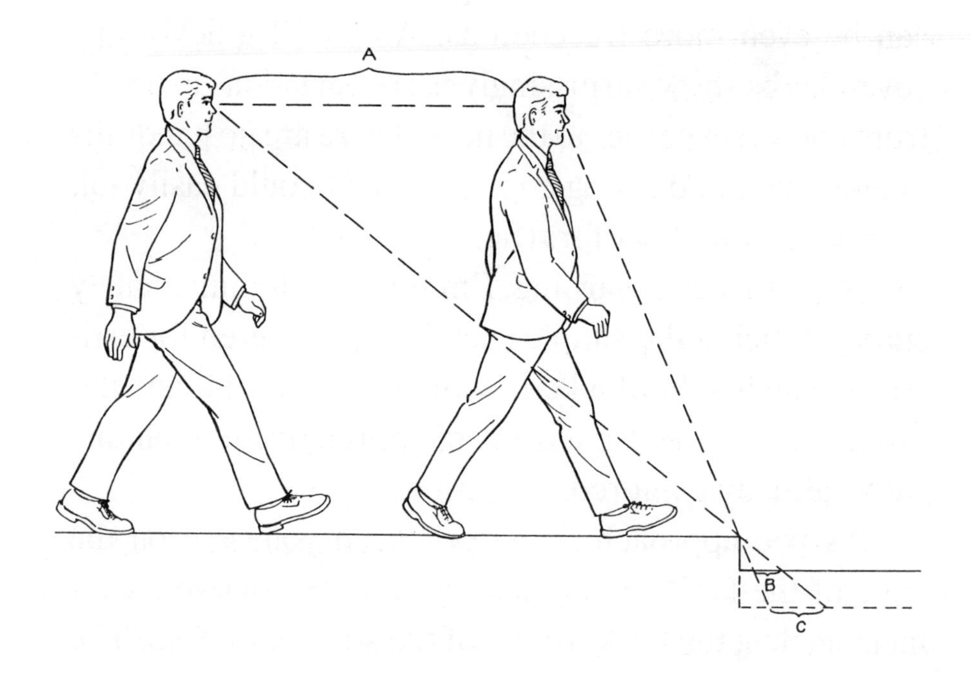

Use the kerb edge as a reference point to judge kerb height. For a low kerb, segment B will be short compared with C for a higher kerb.

Crossing Roads

Now that I've got you to the kerb, I'd better alert you to the dangers out there on the street itself. You're well aware, I'm sure, of the dangers traffic poses for a pedestrian with two good eyes. But the special hazard for the one-eyed is the car that comes from an unexpected quarter on your wrong side. The only way to cope, of course, is to develop the habit of looking both ways *at the very last moment* — and particularly on the side with limited peripheral vision.

Beware of crossroads where cars are permitted to make right and left turns. That car that wasn't signaling when you last looked may be turning any
way. Even if you have the right of way, the driver may assume that you'll see him and step aside.

A special danger is the one-way street you haven't been alerted to — especially if you have a left-side visual cutoff and the traffic is moving from that quarter. If you assume you are crossing a normal two-way street and look first to your right, you might easily step off the kerb into the path of a car bearing down on your left.

A particularly vicious form of this danger awaits the one-eyed visitor from Great Britain going to a country where the motorists drive on the right or vice versa. Busy crossings in London have signs on the pavement reminding you to "Look Right," but elsewhere in this nation it's all too easy for a visitor to step into a lethal situation.

(Ed. Note.) A situation I know all too well. My

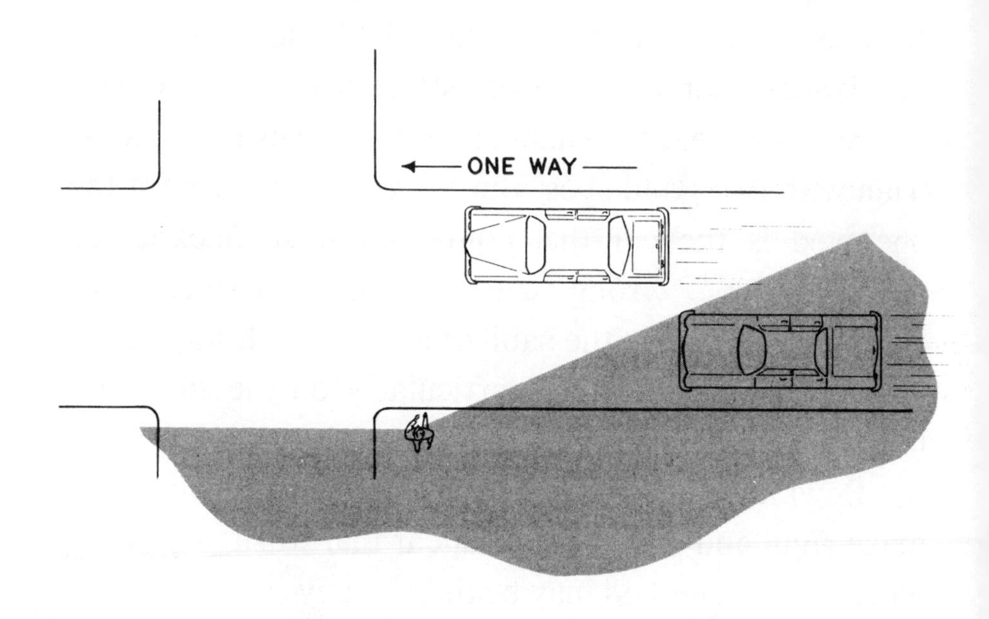

Always be sure to take a good look both ways before stepping off any kerb into the street. But as illustrated above, particular care is necessary when crossing one-way streets.

daughter who lived in Britain for several years was constantly reminding me "Dad, look right, look right." It's a good thing she did as there were several times I would have been the ornament on the front of a London taxi, if I had not heeded her reminders.

Once you have lost your, binocular vision, the best advice anyone can give you for making it to the other side of the road is: *Think before you act.*.

Threading a Needle

This simple act, when first attempted with one eye, can

seem as exasperatingly difficult as trying to pin the tail on the donkey with both eyes blindfolded. Don't rage, don't despair. Here's a technique that works:

1. Cut the thread at an angle with a very sharp pair of scissors or a razor blade. Make sure there's no fuzz on the end. The thread will now have a definite point at the end you've cut.

2. Sharpen that point by moistening it and drawing it between your fingers.

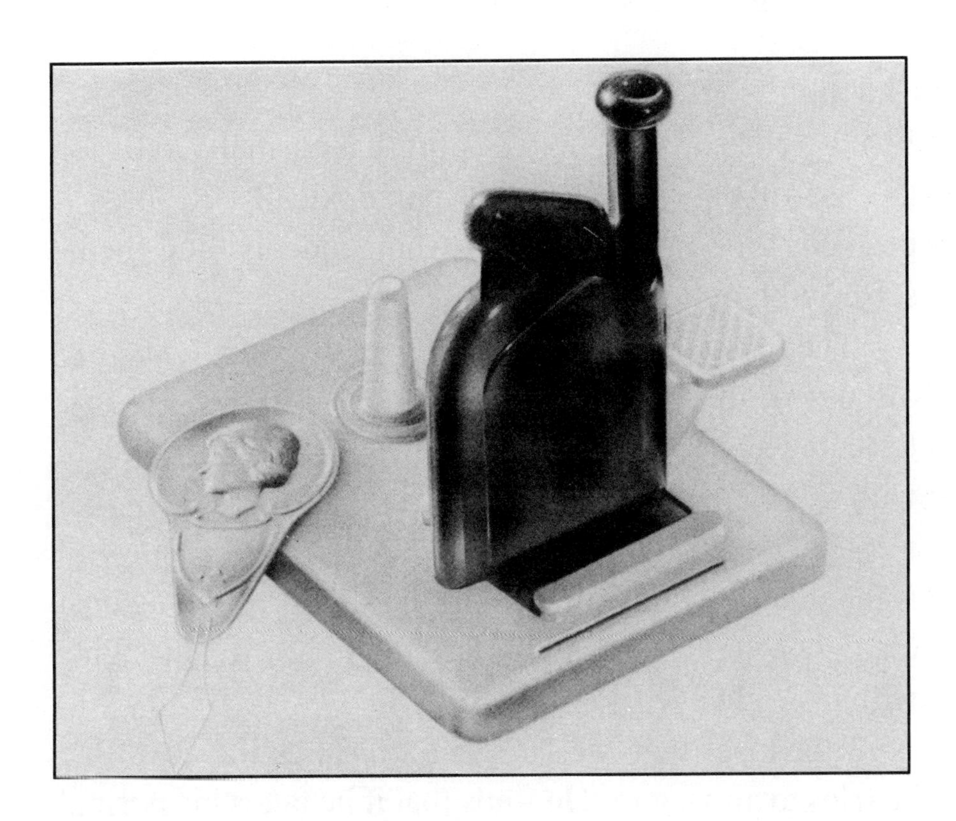

Two common needle-treading devices.

3. Hold the needle toward the light and wipe the point of the thread back and forth across the needle, slowly withdrawing it until it just doesn't touch. The trick is to get the point as close as possible to the eye before the final step.

4. Now centre the point of the thread on the eye of the needle and push it through.

However, a simple needle-threading device such as you can buy in a Woolworth's or a similar store will make the job considerably easier — especially if you also apply the techniques listed above.

Shooting

Firing a rifle or shotgun is a sport that normally calls for the use of only one eye. Yet paradoxically, it poses a problem for some marksmen who suddenly find themselves with only one eye.

The reason is not abstruse. It lies in the fact, already discussed, that right-handed people are right-eyed, and left-handed people left-eyed. This creates no problem with side arms — the difficulty arises only with guns that must be braced against the shoulder. The marksman with right-side dominance normally holds the stock against his right shoulder, places his left foot forward, and sights with his right eye.

If he loses that eye, he's in for a shock the next time he tries to aim a gun. He finds that if he takes his normal stance and holds the weapon against his right shoulder, the gunstock prevents his left eye from lining up with the sights. And a person who loses a dominant left eye, of course, faces the same problem in reverse.

The most common, perhaps the best way, to cope with this problem (though I'll give you some alternatives in Chapter 12) is "switching." This means simply reversing your stance and holding the gun against the other shoulder so you can line up the sights with your remaining good eye.

The first time you try this, everything will feel all wrong. Your scores will show a dramatic drop, particularly if you're shooting at a live or moving target. It'll never work, you'll quickly conclude. Yet many people who'd rather switch than fight have with persistence brought their scores back up to their old levels.

One enthusiastic advocate of switching is my friend Jack Fletcher, a photographic specialist with the National Geographic Society. An avid skeet fan, Jack had been shooting for years without ever having achieved a perfect score. Then he lost his dominant right eye and had to find an instructor to teach him how to shoot off his left shoulder. The training was so successful, that Jack has since shot not one but several perfect scores.

ONE PRECAUTION: Guns with automatic ejection devices are designed to eject the shells away from the person who is firing — and most of them are for shooting off thc right shoulder. Switching could cause the shell to fly toward you and create a hazard. Be sure to keep this problem in mind when you select your firearms.

Exercise

Practically all the skills called for in the simple acts of everyday living with one eye can be sharpened by exercising with a ball. Simply bouncing a ball off a wall for a few minutes each day or playing catch with a friend can improve your visual skills enormously. So can any of the ball games like tennis, cricket, or basketball.

All these activities demand adjustment and call for judgment of angle size, distance, relative motion, and timing. And all the gains you make in these activities can be carried over into your daily routines.

10 In the Driver's Seat

There's no reason why, under normal circumstances, you can't learn or continue to drive with only one eye. (Chapter 15, "Driver and Pilot Licensing Standards," gives specific information concerning licensing requirements.) But there are a few situations in driving that you may find a bit bothersome and that will require some special attention.

I'm sure you'll have no more trouble than I did on the motorway. Actually, most of your visual problems will be on narrow, crowded streets, and at times when you're driving slowly and trying to judge distances on either side of you.

One difficult feat, until you're accustomed to monocular vision, is threading your way through a narrow lane between parked cars without scraping any paint off them. Three ways to handle this (in increasing order of difficulty) are:

• Follow the car ahead of you. With this "guinea pig" to tell you if it's safe to proceed, you'll have no problem (unless you're driving a Bentley and following a Mini.)

• If there's no car ahead of you, then *press your passenger into service* to assure clearance on the left while you concentrate on the right.

• If you have no passenger, *look ahead to make sure you have adequate clearance, and concentrate all your attention to driving close to the line of cars on your right* with your head out the window if necessary.

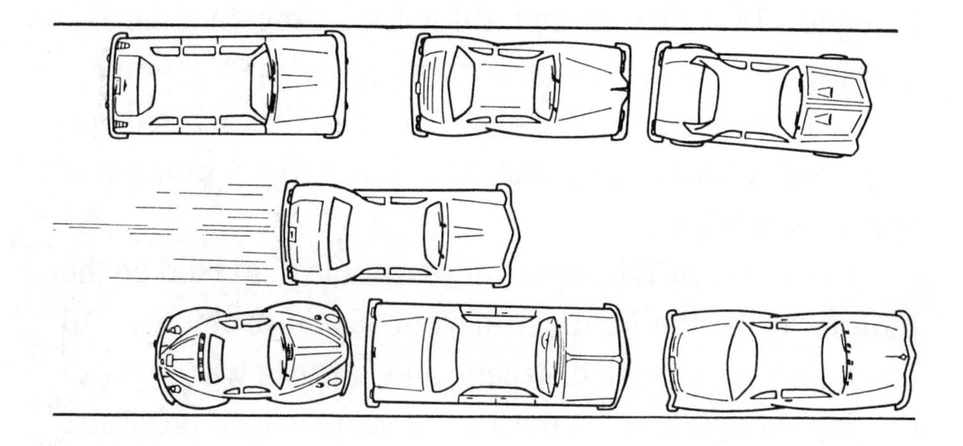

Until you get used to monocular vision you'll probably have trouble working your way between parked cars on a narrow street. Tip: Keep right!

A more nerve-twanging variant of this is the narrow two-way street where you have to make room for an oncoming car without touching the cars parked to your left. Your three alternatives in this problem are:

• Drive close to the centre line so as to leave plenty of room between yourself and the parked cars.

• If there is no centre line, *project a "mental" one onto the street* and try to use it the same way.

• If this proves too difficult, *stop your car at the widest available space* and wait for him to pass.

Car safety engineers could make a real contribution by requiring the corner posts on all new cars be designed to minimize visual obstruction. The wide posts so popular on some cars today can block out an astonishingly large swath of the scene to the rear, even for a driver with good binocular vision. When sight is limited to one eye, the problem is severely aggravated, and the only antidote I know is a limber neck. Frequent head movements will enable you to see around the obstruction and avert any compromise with safety.

Parking

One of the things you sooner or later must learn is to accept your limitations. If you know what you can't do, you may save yourself a lot of pain and frustration by trying to avoid certain situations altogether.

Consider parking. Before my accident, I prided myself on my deftness in parking a car. So it took some ulcerating experimentation to convince me that I'm just not adept anymore. I find that manoeuvring my car into a tight space in a car park lot between two other cars — and knowing that the slightest bump can result in costly damage, thanks to incredibly bad car design — is often more aggravation that it's worth.

If there's a passenger with me, I have no hesitancy about putting him to work to help me clear the other cars. When I'm alone, I sometimes get out of my car to survey the situation and plan my manoeuvres with precision. But more often, if there's time, I'll try to find a wider space or even go considerably out of my way to find a spot I can get into and out of with ease.

Maybe parking will be easy for you. I often marvel at the aplomb of a garage attendant in my office building. While wearing a patch over one eye, this young man races the cars through underground labyrinths, jockeying this one and that one from rear to front, all with the greatest assurance and enjoyment. Whether his monocular vision has anything to do with the dents and scratches customers claim they sometimes find on their cars, I'm not in a position to say. But I wish I knew the secret of his assurance.

I *have* developed a trick or two that you can use for snuggling into your own garage without hitting the rear wall. Turn on the headlights, even in the daytime and watch the patterns the beams make on the wall as you approach it. In no time, you will be able to come within an inch and not hit. At night, you can also back in and use the rear lights in the same manner.

Another very simply and effective aid is a short strip of tape pasted vertically on the sidewall of the garage adjacent to your good eye to mark your stopping point. I find that my garage parking, using this technique, is much more uniform and accurate than that of other drivers in my family who rely solely on depth perception.

I have a friend, Stu Chapman, who, when he gets a new car, slowly parks the new car so that the bumper just touches the wall of his garage. He then makes a simple wooden frame 3″ longer than the distance from the wall to the tyres which he places on the floor of the garage. All he has to do when parking, is to drive slowly until he feels the resistance of the frame and he is safely parked 3″ from the wall.

CHOOSING A NEW CAR

When you are in the market for a new car, you will want to consider several features that are more important to you than the average car buyer. They are field of vision, size and all-weather capability.

For visibility, check whether the car's design allows you to see all around. Do corner posts obstruct your view and does curved glass distort what you see? Do you sit high enough to see over the bonnet and boot? Does the inside rear view mirror give you a wide angle view?

New cars are now equipped with quartz halogen headlights which provide far more illumination than sealed beam units. If you're not in the market for a new car, and won't be for a while, you can get quartz lamps for your present car. For a further discussion, see the Driving Aids section of Chapter 12.

Your car's size makes a big difference for driving ease. If you've been driving a large car, test-drive a small one and see how much extra room you have for parking or manoeuvring through tight traffic. You may find driving a lot more fun.

While defrosters, windscreen wipers, "squirt" windscreen washers and rear window defoggers are standard equipment, if you do much bad-weather driving you may find it worthwhile to have a rear-window washer/wiper as well. They can add a lot to your peace of mind.

There is no reason why you can't safely drive a minimally equipped car, but driving one with the features I've described above can increase your comfort and enjoyment. And, with a car like this in bad weather, you'll be able to see more with your one eye than most of the drivers on the road.

11 The Active Life

Anyone who feels that the loss of an eye marks the end of taking part in sports activities should consider the case of Sue Moran, radio and TV personality, fashion model, committeewoman, and mother of six. Mrs. Moran's 10-year bout with a corneal inflammation ended with the loss of her right eye.

"It hasn't changed my life," she says. "I'm still doing all the things I enjoy and still coping with the endless demands that come with a large family and a country home."

Among the things Mrs. Moran enjoys is riding in such competitions as the International Horse Show in Washington, where she has won a reputation for her skill in the vanishing art of riding sidesaddle. She also enjoys fox hunting, beagling, swimming, skiing, and bird watching — all sports that make heavy demands on visual perception and judgment.

Because the speeds involved demand lightning judgments, skiing would seem to require the ultimate in visual perception. Yet ski-jumper Jerry Martin from Minnesota has proved that top-level, competitive skiing is really possible with one eye.

Martin lost the sight in his right eye in September 1971, when a nail he was pounding into brick bounced back and struck his cornea. Six weeks after his injury, he was jumping again. And he was doing it so well that by January 1972 he won the tryouts for the U.S. Olympic team with a leap of 318 feet. (He failed to win a medal at the Olympics, but he did place higher than any other American.)

Commenting on his winning tryout performance, Martin said: "My doctor told me depth perception would be the biggest problem. In ski jumping you need it for taking off and for landing, but you're only affected at a distance of about 10 feet. I've been jumping a long time and I land more by feel than by sight, so I wasn't worried about that. I wanted to prove to myself that I could keep jumping with one eye. That actually gave me a little extra push."

In contrast, Sandy Duncan, brilliant TV comedy star who lost the sight in one eye, gave a magazine reported an hilarious account of her efforts to learn to ski. Time after time, while standing and talking with her instructor, she'd suddenly find herself starting to slide down the slope: "Finally, we figured it out. Because of this eye thing I can't determine the fall line. I would think I was exactly on the perpendicular when in fact I was headed straight down the slope." But with the same determination she's shown in coping with her handicap, Miss Duncan added, "I'll learn."

As you test yourself out in the sports that have always given you pleasure, there are a few important physical and psychological factors to keep in mind. From a purely physical standpoint, those sports in which the motion takes place in two dimensions rather than three — bowling, billiards, croquet, and shuffleboard, for example — will be the easiest to remaster. Since the object of play is confined to a single plane, the simple visual judgments demanded in these sports can be handled with one eye just about as well as with two.

In three-dimensional sports, where monocular vision presents more of a challenge, your difficulties will be determined by many more factors. A basketball, for instance, will be easier to manage than a handball; you'll miss less often with a racket than with a bat; a fast game like jai alai will come a lot harder than a slower one like badminton.

Squash is a fast game, but you'll be able to play it. Before you do, though, let me give you a special word of warning. This increasingly popular walled-court sport accounts for a number of eye injuries far out of proportion to the number of its participants. I don't condemn the sport and say it should be avoided, but whoever plays it should know the risks involved and take suitable precautions. A U.S. Navy publication reports that 75 Navy men suffered squash-related eye injuries during the years

1970 to 1976. The U.S. Air Force count of accidents on walled-courts included 25 eye injuries and one fatality. The risk of injury is so great that in September 1978 Canada passed a law that requires squash players to wear eye guards.

Players with normal vision ought to wear non-prescription industrial safety glasses or other suitable protective eyewear. A player with only one eye shouldn't venture onto a court without the best eye protection available. Regular prescription glasses with impact-resistant lenses can help somewhat in case of an accident, but aren't nearly as effective as industrial glasses or the "combat glasses" described in the next chapter. And in this case, even the best is not good enough.

But given the right psychological set, no sport is beyond the capabilities of the person who has lost an eye. Nor is there any reason to give up those that have always brought you enjoyment. The main thing to remember is that some sports call for a longer period of relearning than others, and that during this period you're competing only with yourself.

This psychological stance may be a little harder to acquire in such games as tennis and cricket, in which the emphasis seems to be entirely on beating an adversary. If you find any of these too frustrating, why not try making your comeback, initially, in sports that have well-established handicaps, like golf? Or those that pit you against your own record, like archery or rifle practice? Or those that you can engage in purely for fun and exercise — as well as for competition when you want it — like water sports?

Water sports, in fact, have so much to recommend them to the newly one-eyed that I'd like to discuss a few of them individually.

Swimming

This most popular of all water sports is virtually unaffected by the limitations of monocular vision. And this is true not only of surface swimming, but of underwater swimming with snorkel or scuba equipment.

Underwater distance judgments are difficult even with normal eyesight because water bends the light differently from the way air does. Moreover, most underwater masks limit the field of vision so much that it makes no difference whether you have one eye or two.

So if this activity appeals to you, it's one of the best ways to get back in the swim.

Diving

You'll encounter no special problems here either, unless you wear an artificial eye. The sudden pressure when you strike the water, particularly in a high dive, can dislodge the prosthesis. A pair of underwater goggles is the answer. To safeguard your good eye, make sure the lenses are high-impact and shatter-resistant.

Fishing

Although some distance judgments are involved in casting a line, the distances are beyond the range where binocular vision is any real help. Out of the Bahama flats I've watched my one-eyed friend Clarke Daniel, with all the skill and precision of a native bonefish guide, drop his shrimp-baited hooks time after time directly in front of bonefish.

The chief danger is having a wild cast put a hook into your eye. Lewis Williams Douglas lost an eye this way while serving as U.S. ambassador in Britain. With only one good eye, you simply can't afford to take that chance, so always wear protective glasses — even if you don't need glasses to correct your vision — with high-impact, shatter-resistant lenses.

Water Skiing and Surfing

These sports, though difficult in themselves, pose absolutely no special problems for the one-eyed individual.

Although if you wear an artificial eye, it is wise to leave it behind. A fall could dislodge it and they are difficult, if not impossible to find at the bottom of a lake. Goggles will protect your good eye and prevent irritation to your socket from water, chlorine, salt, etc. While they will also help prevent loss of your prosthesis, I feel that it is better to be overcautious and remove it and then put on goggles before indulging in water sports.

Sailing

Just a few points for the newly-monocular to remember. The danger in jumping from dock to boat or vice versa can be lessened by following the old sailors advice "One hand for the boat."

Ed. Note: Three months after failing to heed this advice, our editor was still removing slivers from his hide because of misjudging the distance between a boat and the dock.

A useful advice for all skippers, but particularly the one-eyed, is the "telltale" — bits of yarn placed on the shrouds or at the luff to indicate the relative direction of the wind and help obtain the proper trim.

A monocle for the checking distant buoys and an illuminated magnifier for reading charts at night are also useful. A "monkey fist," or padded weight at the end of a small line, can improve your accuracy when you toss a line to shore or to another boat. Ingenious devices like these can more than compensate for the limitations of monocular vision. In the next chapter, we'll talk about other devices you'll find helpful.

Meanwhile, I'd like to give a plug for one non-athletic activity that people with severely impaired vision can participate in on equal terms with others — amateur radio. Operating, whether voice or code, depends primarily on the hearing and touch.

It's fairly easy to get on the air with a novice class license. You can get whatever information you need to, pass the licence exam by writing to:

FA42
Radio Amateur Licence Unit
Chetwynd House

Chesterfield
Derbyshire
S49 1PF
Telephone 0246-216-555

They will provide you with details of their licence requirements in the booklet "How to Become a Radio Amateur".

If you're already on the air or if you get your ticket, be sure to give me a call. I'm W3MSB and currently operate CW (code) only.

12 Gimmicks and Gadgets - Let Technology Help

How do you turn a handicap into an asset?

One way is by taking full advantage of all the marvellous gadgetry created to compensate — even overcompensate — for every imaginable deficiency. Many people deprived of binocular vision have found that one eye plus a gadget plus a little practice results in a better performance than had been thought possible with two eyes unaided. So let's examine some of the aids and instruments you may find helpful.

Spectacles

When you've lost one eye, it becomes imperative to protect the surviving one and to enhance its vision to the greatest practicable degree. Of course, only an eye specialist can tell you whether you need glasses and prescribe the proper corrective lens for you. But there are some special considerations to keep in mind when you go to get his prescription filled. There've been quite a few developments in eye glasses since Ben Franklin invented bifocals in the 18th century.

Some of the most effective developments in eye safety have been the safety standards set by the British Standards Institution, requiring all Industrial Safety glasses sold in the U.K. to be impact resistant. As a result, almost 100% of the spectacles for industrial use are made from polycarbonate resins.

Impact resistance for industrial plano (non-prescription) eyeglasses means that a grade 1 lens must be able to withstand, without breaking, the impact of a 6.35mm steel ball propelled onto the surface of the lens at a velocity of 120m/s per second.

At present, about 40% of prescription lenses are made of polycarbonate and about 50% out of CR-39 Optical Plastic. The balance is produced with heat or chemically hardened glass lenses. There is no standard for prescription lenses at the moment. However new standards are expected to be issued just after the time this book is printed.

Because of their lightness and thinness, the use of polycarbonate lenses is growing every year, even though the surface of the lens may be scratched more easily despite its scratch resistant coating.

Special lenses for sports activities such as racquet sports, hockey, basketball, or skiing are made from polycarbonate to the industrial standard.

If in your work or hobbies (like woodworking or gardening) there is a possibility of material flying around your face, I suggest the addition of clear side shields which are available from your optician or safety supply store.

My suggestion, based on experience, even if you do not require glasses for vision improvement, is to buy a pair with polycarbonate lenses with no corrective grinding. Possibly with a slight tint at the top of the lens but certainly not all over. (See note re Sandy Duncan in Chapter 14). You will have enough to do in learning to cope with this new lifestyle. The concerns you will have in protecting your remaining vision will, at times, border on paranoia. Don't worry about it as it is a very real and normal reaction.

However, help make the adjustment easier on yourself by acquiring a little bit of extra protection which will provide some assurance and will, at least in your mind, reduce the feeling of being conspicuous. Because, in truth you really are not different and most people are not aware of a physical change in you. Here endeth the sermon.

Your visual field, as you know, has already been reduced, and for some activities you certainly won't want to cut it down any more. So choose spectacle styles accordingly. Glasses with heavy frames, for instance, may be fine for reading, but they cut off so much of your field that they constitute a severe — and totally unnecessary — handicap when you're driving a car, watching a cricket match, or engaging in any other activity that calls for a panoramic view.

Thin-rimmed or rimless glasses cut this problem to a minimum, and a contact lens eliminates it altogether.

The crescent-shaped half glasses that many people use for reading are also good in this respect, since you get an unobstructed view over the top of the lens.

Wire frame glasses don't reduce your visual field excessively, but they may be dangerous if you wear them while playing sports. If the glasses receive a hard blow, the sharp wire can severely damage an eye. There have been reports of this type of accident. Today, there are many models of rimless glasses available from most manufac-

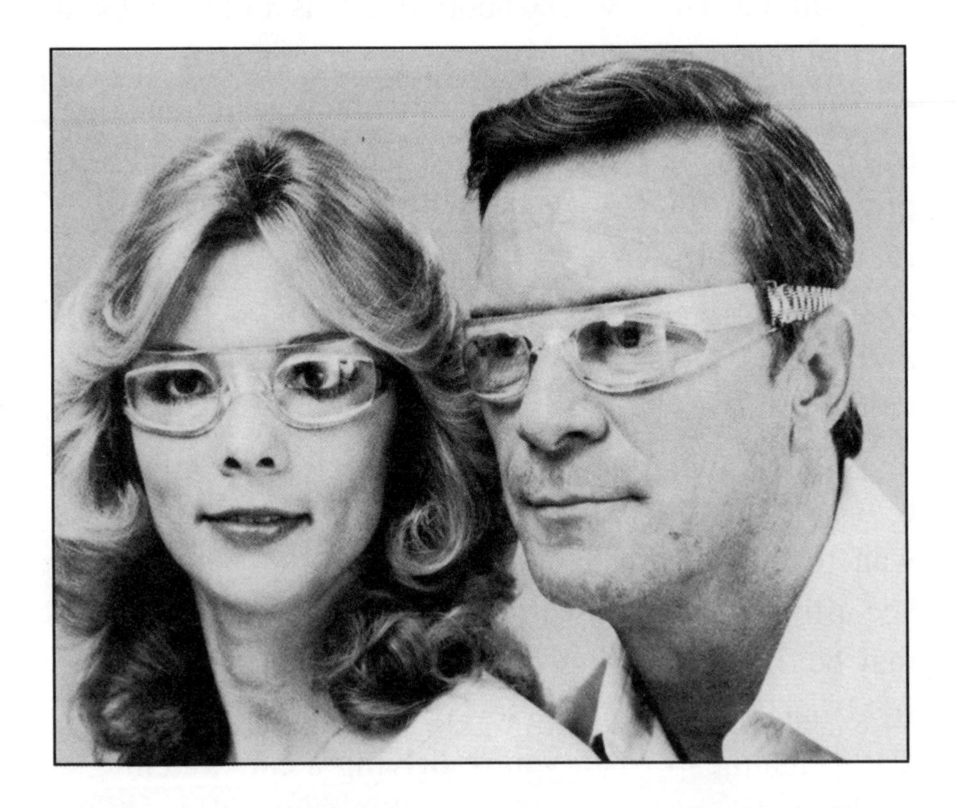

Combat glasses, designed specifically for protection in active sports, have a particular advantage for the one-eyed. The wraparound design allows for the widest possible range of vision.

turers. The lens is held in a groove in the circumference of the lens by a tough nylon thread. At no point does the glass touch metal. The result is a strong construction with minimum obstruction to peripheral vision.

However, rimless glasses are not included in safety glass design since they do not hold the lens securely enough. Even with the nylon cord, the lens could dislodge or move back during the impact and could strike the eye.

A positive (plus) lens prescription provides a thinner edge thickness although the centre thickness is greater. A minus lens prescription is thicker at the edge.

There are special frames for sportsmen, featuring a headband that keeps them from being knocked off — a type any yachtsman who has ever lost a pair of glasses overboard appreciates greatly. (Floating frames are another solution to this problem.)

What is generally acknowledged, by many experts, as the best designed and produced eyewear for sports was developed in Canada by Imperial Optical Company. These glasses are designed specifically to provide protection in active sports, such as hockey, football, squash, baseball and cricket.

Their Khan II model is being exported to many nations including the U.S. and U.K. A major sports equipment manufacturer is selling tens of thousands of pairs a year in the U.S. This frame has a tough plastic wrap around body with adjustable headband, and they take prescription lenses. They can also be used on jobs that present hazards to the eyes. A particular advantage for the monocular is

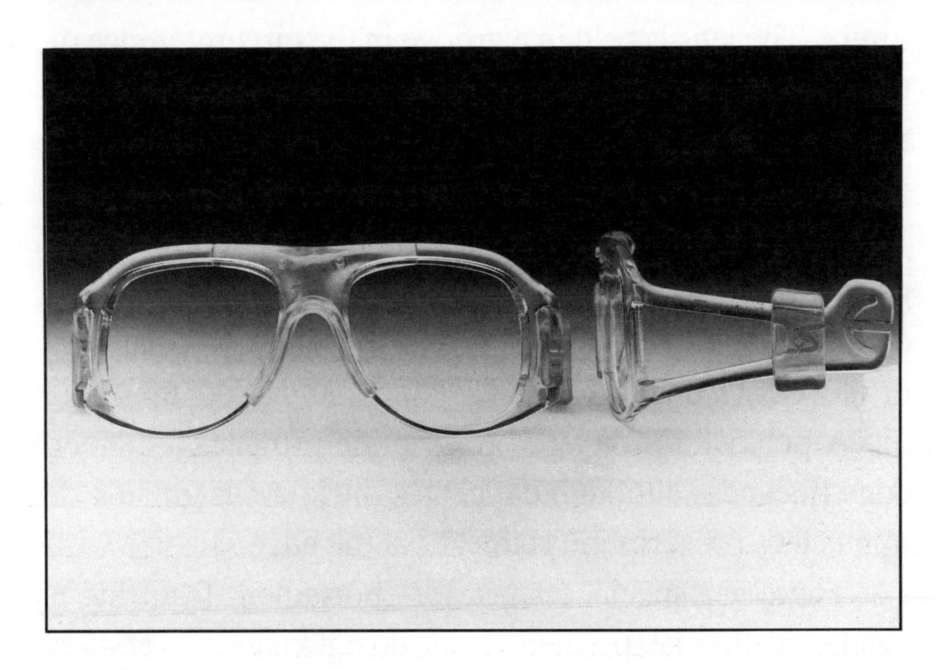

their wrap around design, which offers an exceptionally wide range of vision.

These high protection glasses are available from many opticians in Britain. To get additional information on where to acquire them call:

Imperial Optical,
30 Alexandra Street,
Southend-on-Sea,
Essex,
SSE 1BW

Telephone: 702 335 520

If this sounds like a testimonial for a particular brand of eyewear, it is. But is is an unpaid testimonial. I have a pair and thcy arc grcat.

You can also choose from a wide variety of lens tints and coatings designed for special purposes. For example, it's advantageous to use a shade of yellow when you're shooting because it absorbs blue light, providing maximum haze penetration.

Some lenses are treated to darken when sunlight hits them, so the wearer needn't change glasses every time he goes out in the sun or comes back indoors. But under certain conditions, these photochromic lenses actually pose a hazard to the wearer. At least one major airline has alerted its pilots to the dangers. First, the shadows inside a car and in an airplane cockpit may not allow the lenses' sensitive material to be activated, and the wearer isn't getting the protection he needs.

A more serious problem is the time it takes photochromic lenses to clear when light conditions change from bright to dim. One test reported that lenses were only 50 per cent clear five minutes after they were removed from sunlight and still only 75 per cent clear after 20 minutes. Some of the lenses never become more than 80 per cent clear, which makes them unsuitable for night driving or flying. Even in the daylight-to-dusk period the lenses don't change fast enough, and unfortunately, this kind of light change is too gradual to warn the wearer that his vision is being impaired.

There is a non-reflective lens coating that not only makes the wearer's eyes more visible to others, but reduces distracting reflections and ghost images. Because most of the light passes through the lens instead of being reflected away, the wearer gets a clearer view. Glasses with this kind of lens are particularly useful for driving.

An optical system for the one-eyed has been developed that extends peripheral vision on the side of the missing eye. I can't report on its effectiveness, because the considerable cost of fitting the lack of any convincing assurance of its advantages discourage me from testing the system.

I mention these developments in eyewear not to recommend some and tell you to avoid others, but to make you aware of them and better able to discuss your particular needs with an ophthalmologist. And remember that whatever type of glasses you're buying — whether for improved vision or protection form the sun or whatever — to safeguard your single precious eye be sure it has non-shatterable lenses that comply with the law.

Just a word that may save you some money when you buy glasses. Many retail suppliers of eyewear allow for the fact that the monocular need only one prescription lens, and they adjust their charges accordingly. Others charge full price. Next time you have a lens prescription filled, don't hesitate to ask for half price. There may not be many advantages to being one-eyed, but this is one of them.

Emergency "Glasses'

Ever get caught in front of a telephone book with no glasses to keep the print from blurring? Here's an emergency measure I picked up somewhere — and have often been thankful for ever since:

Take a small piece of cardboard or paper — a calling card is fine — and punch a tiny hole in it with a pin or a bent paper clip (the lead in an automatic lead pencil will also do nicely). Now place your eye against the hole, hold the small print about six inches from your eye — and read. What you've got is a lens that operates on the same principle as Grandfather's pinhole camera. You may not want to read *Gone With the Wind* this way, but it works in an emergency.

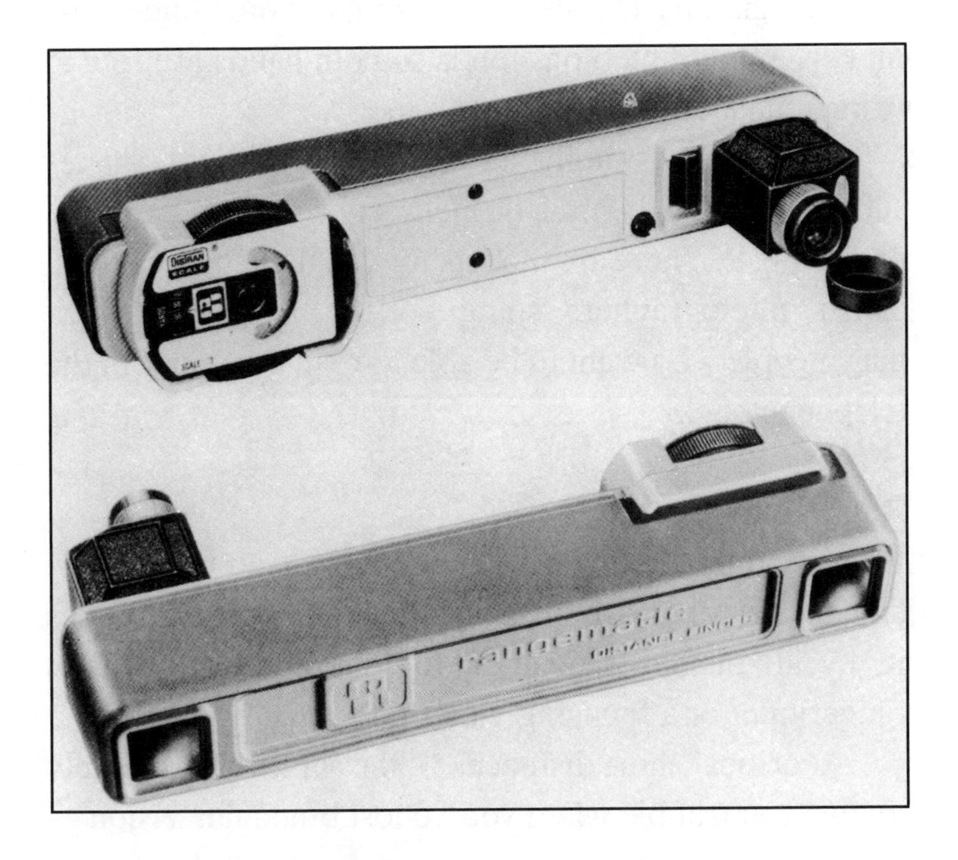

Rangefinders are invaluable aids in determining distances. The model shown here works on the stereopsis (coincidence of images) principle.

Magnifiers

The loss of an eye can become much more of a problem if vision deteriorates in the surviving eye. One kind of deterioration affecting many adults is a decreasing ability to focus on near objects. In the one-eyed, this can easily reach a point where even corrective glasses are inadequate for reading small print or doing close work.

A magnifying glass can often solve the problem, and there's a wide selection available, ranging from small pocket versions to large desk units. Some industrial models are mounted on stands so both hands are free to work beneath the glass.

Many units combine a magnifier and a light source, such as a torch behind the lens or a fluorescent tube encircling it. There are models for yachtsmen, jewellers, artists, photographers, stamp collectors, and just ordinary people who want to be able to read a number in the telephone book.

Rangefinders

If your camera is the kind that requires you to estimate how far away you are from your subject in order to focus it, by all means trade it in for one equipped with a rangefinder or a focusing viewfinder.

At critical short distances — the same that are likely to give you trouble when you've lost binocular vision — your camera requires more exact focus; and a rangefinder or a focusing viewfinder will give you far better results than you ever got by estimating, even when you

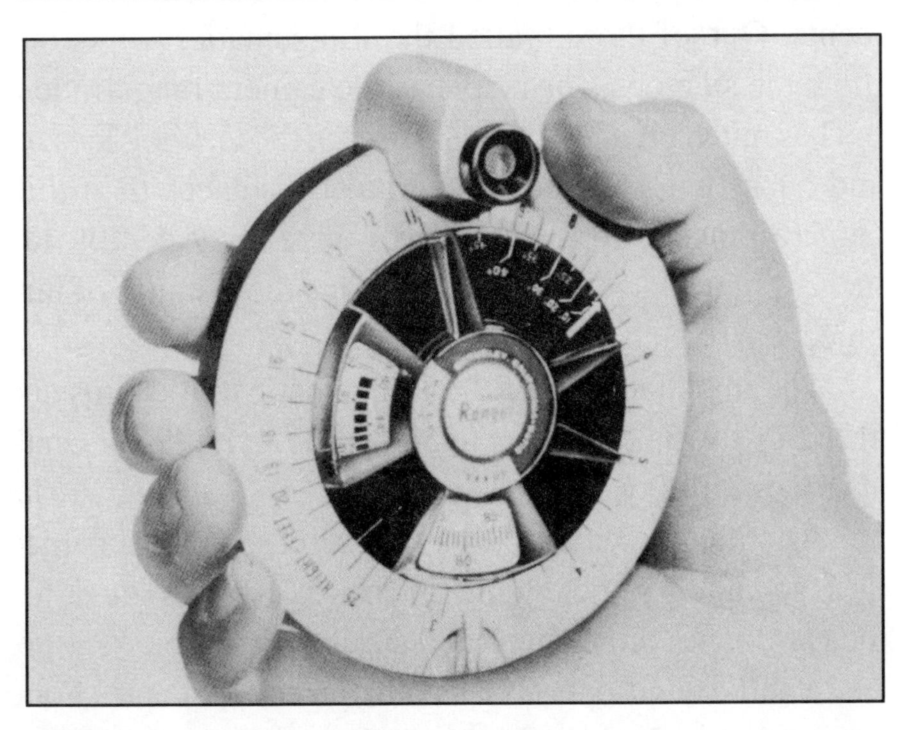

This compact, stadimetric rangefinder depends on knowing the length or height of an object.

had two good eyes.

An exciting development in photography is the introduction of automatic-focusing cameras that allow the user to simply point and shoot. Clever almost beyond belief, one of these, the Polaroid, is based on a sonar principle. A little chirp emitted by the camera bounces off the subject and back to the camera. The camera focuses itself on the basis of how long it takes for the sound to travel.

Several rangefinders on the market are useful to hunters, fishermen, yachtsmen, golfers and others who have a need for reasonably accurate distance measurements. One of these, called the Rangematic, works on the same stereopsis principle as the camera rangefinder but has much greater spacing between the viewing lenses and hence can be used over greater distances than the camera rangefinders. If our eyes were separated by 10 inches, we would also be able to judge the distance of far objects more accurately.

The manufacturer of the Rangematic unit claims an accuracy of 95 per cent up to 500 yards and a 99 per cent accuracy at 100 yards.

Another device that uses the stereoscopic principle is a so-called optical tape measure. It's designed to measure room dimensions and similar distances.

Another unit operates on a different principle. You need only to select an object of known height or length, set two dials, and read the distance from a scale. For example, knowing the height of the flag on a golf green, a player would simply set the dials, read off the distance, and finally select the right club for his shot.

In golf as well as other activities requiring distance judgments, the one-eyed player is at a disadvantage only when it comes to short distances. The rangefinders described above might be highly useful to persons with normal binocular vision.

Other Optical Aids

Many gadgets are available for raising your eyepower. If you search the optical-goods market, you'll find a wide variety of instruments made to be used with one eye —

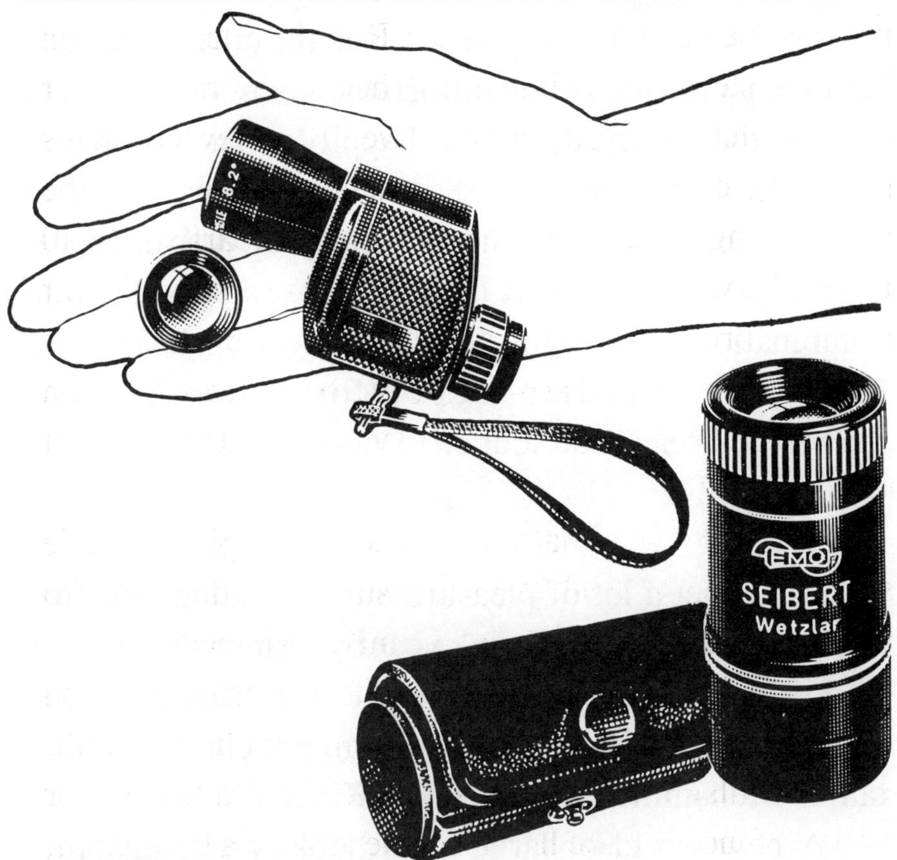

Two handy, hand-sized viewers.
Above: a combination telescope and magnifier.
Below: telescope/miscoscope unit.

telescopes, microscopes, loupes, and monocles, to name a few examples.

People with normal binocular vision sometimes have difficulty getting accustomed to these instruments, because there's always the problem of "What'll I do with the other eye?" Students who must use single lens microscopes for long periods are taught to keep both eyes open — and it usually takes them quite a while before they're no longer distracted by what the unused eye is seeing.

Closing that eye for long periods, on the other hand, can become increasingly uncomfortable.

For the one-eyed, there is happily no such problem. You'll find any one of these instruments easy to use at first try and, if it's well made, highly effective. Moreover, if you like this sort of thing, you can buy them in combinations to delight your gadgeteering heart — a telescope-magnifier-loupe, for instance, or a microscope-telescope-loupe.

Large Print

If you get a lot of pleasure out of reading, but find that the type seems to shrink year by year so that glasses no longer do the job, then maybe it is time you tried something new. Here is what you might call the mountain to Mohammed approach: BIGGER TYPE

A new world of large-print books and magazines awaits you, ranging from ancient history to modern cookbooks, from Homer to Hemingway. Children's books, maps, song sheets, and crossword puzzles are now available, and new material is being added all the time. Most local public libraries stock a selection of large-print books.

The best source of information regarding large print books that I have seen is the pamphlet "Some Sources of Large Print Material" distributed by the Royal National Institute for the Blind. Their Address is:

224 Great Portland Street
London

W1N 6AA
Phone 071 338 1266

Among the references given is:
LARGE TYPE BOOKS IN PRINT
Published by R.R. Bowker (UK)
This book lists over 6000 titles published by over 70 publishers.

One organization that provides help and support to the newly monocular is: The Partially Sighted Society
Queen's Road
Doncaster
South Yorkshire
DN1 2NX

Their support over the years in providing the Original U.S. edition of "A Singular View" is greatly appreciated.

There is a 40 page weekly news summary published that includes a complete listing of the next week's radio and television programmes. It is available by quarterly or annual subscription from:
BIG PRINT LIMITED
P.O. Box 308
Warrington
Cheshire
WA1 1JE

They have a great offer. Send them a letter and they will send you a FREE copy as a trial before you sub scribe. Sounds like a good deal to me.

Many banks including Barclays, Lloyds, Midland, and National Westminster will provide large-print statements for their clients. Enquire at your branch.

British Telecom has a large-print dial which fits over the existing dial of a telephone. Contact the sales division of your local manager's office.

Measuring Tools

It's the little distances that get you down, remember? The inches, feet, and yards or metres, centimetres and millimetres. So keep an extra-generous supply of ordinary measuring tools near at hand — tape measures, yardsticks, rulers, and carpenter's rules. Being forced to make exact measurements instead of guessing will bring the blessings of precision into many jobs you perhaps once didn't do nearly so neatly and nicely.

Lighting

I strongly believe that special kinds of lighting can do much to compensate for the impairments in vision, but other than my own experience I have little evidence to back me up. Much work has been done in studying special lighting requirements of the aged, but I found nothing directed toward the special problems of monocular vision.

Lighting for *normal* vision, by contrast, has been the subject of a great many studies. As a result of this research, lighting engineers always strive for uniform, shadowless light wherever work is done that demands close, critical inspection.

I do a lot of close work myself, and I've found, since losing an eye, that this kind of shadowless light, such as you get from rows and rows of fluorescent tubes, is far from satisfactory for really critical tasks. I much prefer a strong, localized light source, such as a small high-intensity lamp, supplemented by a lower level of general illumination. The sharp, definite shadows produced by a high-intensity lamp can be put to excellent use in gauging depth and distance.

Let me give you an example. A small light source mounted close to the work table of a drill-press can be adjusted to cast a sharp shadow of the drill onto the work. As the drill is lowered, the shadow indicates just where the point will touch, and the work can be moved so that the point of the drill will meet its mark precisely. And this same principle can be used in the kitchen, the office, the den — wherever exactness counts.

In the absence of any more scientific evidence than my own say-so, I suggest that you experiment with various combinations of lights, adjusting the angles and distances until you find the arrangement that seems best for the task at hand.

Driving Aids

Two common, inexpensive car accessories I've found useful are a set of kerb feelers and an extra side mirror. The four wire feelers attached to the sides of your car to tell you when you're within inches of the kerb can take the guesswork out of street parking.

A second external mirror mounted on the left side of the car helps not so much in viewing as it does in checking your clearance on that side, particularly at slow speeds, as when you're pulling into your garage or snaking between parked cars.

On the more expensive side — but for safety's sake well worth the cost — are replacements for your headlights. If you're traveling at 55 miles an hour, your standard headlights won't illuminate the whole distance it will take for you to come to a complete stop. The

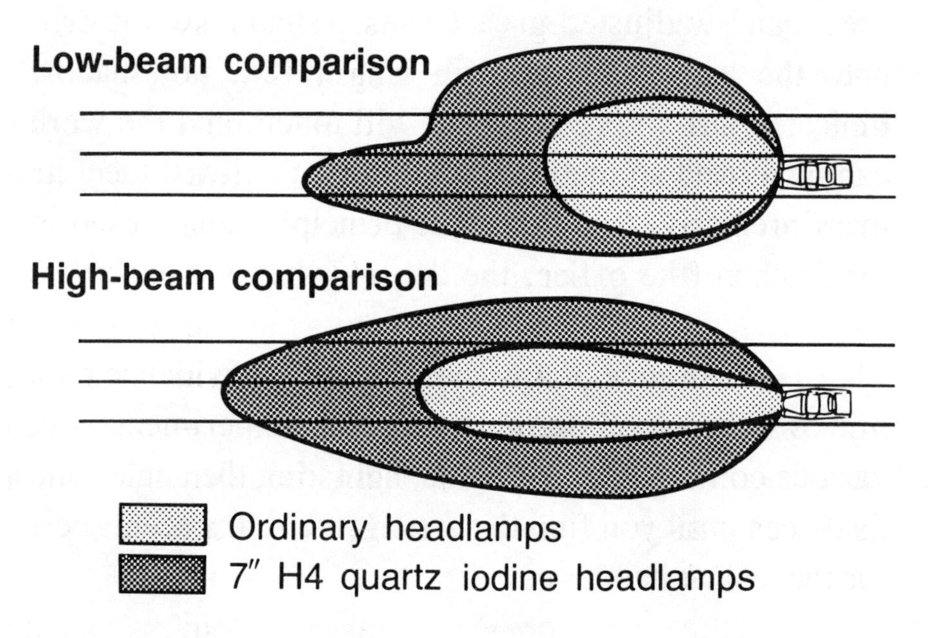

Quartz iodine headlights cover a greater distance and wider range than ordinary headlights. They have lenses that, in low-beam operation, are designed to cast a flat beam away from the eyes of oncoming drivers and still provide almost incredible visibility.

situation is worse, of course, on rainy nights. And the beam they throw is altogether too narrow. These restrictions on your already restricted vision make night driving nerve-wracking.

You can replace your ordinary headlights with quartz iodine or quartz halogen units at a very reasonable cost to more than double your vision ahead and to the sides. The result will be greater safety, of course, and also greater confidence in taking the road at night.

Gun Gadgetry

For the serious marksman who's lost his dominant eye, the best way of regaining his skill is switching — reversing his stance and shooting from the other shoulder. But the training required for this changeover demands considerable time and effort — more than you may wish to devote to it if you're just a casual, now-and-then sort of hunter or marksman like me.

An alternative way of accomplishing the same result is to use a gun with an offset stock. I experimented with one such weapon during a visit to London — a shotgun designed to be fired off the right shoulder, but with a stock that allowed enough head movement to align the left eye with the sights.

In spite of its odd appearance, I found this gun handled very naturally. I was able to shoulder, aim, and fire it quite comfortably — and with no perceptible loss of skill — the very first time I tried it. In fact it seemed to be a very good solution to the problem. Such guns are made to order by Cogswell and Harrison, Ltd.

I have heard that there are also guns with offset sights designed to accomplish the same purpose as offset stocks, but my inquiries to firearms manufacturers have failed to locate one.

In any case, it's evident that with the options available, no hunter or marksman need be afraid that the loss of an eye — even the dominant eye — will interfere with his shooting. Of course, if the dominant eye is the surviving one, there's no problem whatever.

13 Keeping the Good Eye Good

The care and safeguarding of eyesight is a matter of concern to everyone. But for the person who has lost one of his eyes, there are two additional special considerations. The first involves the question of what to do about the nonseeing eye or — if that's been removed — the empty socket. The other consideration is the overriding importance of protecting whatever eyesight remains in the surviving eye.

To get the best advice on eye care for the one-eyed, I consulted Dr. John W. McTigue, chief of the department of ophthalmology of the Washington Medical Center and a distinguished researcher in this field. In the course of our interviews, he became so enthusiastic about my project that he agreed to grace it with a foreword. The fruits of those interviews are contained in this chapter, on which he has so generously collaborated.

This material has subsequently been updated by

some of the staff at Moorfields Eye Hospital to ensure that we used the proper U.K. terminology.

The Eye That Was

If your damaged eye has been removed by surgery (enucleated), care of the remaining socket is usually very simple. Should you decide on a "glass eye" for cosmetic reasons, make sure it's well fitted by an expert; a poorly fitted shell can irritate the conjunctiva, the mucous membrane that lines the eyelid. This or any other irritation of the socket — from infections, foreign bodies, etc. — is usually not serious, provided you have it treated promptly by an ophthalmologist.

The socket may surprise you by continuing to perform many of the functions of a normal eye socket, such as blinking, winking, and even shedding tears, since the lids and tear glands are still in working order.

If you still have your nonseeing eye, the amount of follow-up medical care it needs may vary from very frequent visits to practically none, depending on what caused the loss of vision. so make certain you understand what your condition requires in this respect. Routine follow-up care is usual in such cases.

Be sure to report to your doctor without delay any new symptoms, such as pain or redness. Don't wait to see what develops!

The Surviving Eye

Don't worry about using up your "good" eye — no

matter what the old wives, males and female, may tell you. Your surviving eye is quite capable of taking on by itself all the visual tasks, no matter how demanding, that were once performed by both eyes together.

If that remaining eye is normal, it probably will require only routine preventive care — an ophthalmological checkup every two years may suffice. Again, be sure to consult your own doctor about this. Moreover, you should report to him at once if you experience any new symptoms, such as redness, blurred vision, pain in the eye, or headaches.

For the one-eyed person there are just a few special questions that relate to glasses, contact lenses, and injuries or diseases of the eye.

Glasses

Even small, subtle changes in vision can become important when you've lost an eye, and you'll probably be much quicker to notice them than you used to be. It may be necessary to test your eyesight for glasses more often now. Some patients need a refraction, as this test is called, as frequently as every four months.

Any blurring in vision may be a sign that you need new glasses. The conditions that cause this blurring — myopia (near sightedness), hyperopia (far sightedness), astigmatism (distorted vision) — can generally be corrected by a compensating lens. And so can the loss of focusing power that comes with age (presbyopia). As the surviving eye loses its elasticity, a bifocal, or even a trifocal lens may become necessary to permit quick and easy shifts in focus.

One blessing of advancing years: The eye generally stabilizes by the age of 55 or 60. After that, you may be relatively free of problems caused by vision changes.

Once again, please do be sure to use safety lenses in your glasses and, if you drive, to avoid heavy frames.

Contact Lenses

For the one-eyed person who needs a corrective lens, the contact can be an inestimable boon — provided that the fit is accurate, that medical supervision is regular, and that the patient is careful to exercise good sense about wearing it.

The great advantage of the contact lens is that it provides the clearest and widest visual field possible — which, of course, is of major importance to the person whose field is reduced by the loss of one eye.

Sometimes, as in extreme cases of myopia or hyperopia, a contact lens is the only way to compensate for the loss of side vision. This is particularly true after the removal of cataracts, when ordinary glasses provide only "tunnel vision," a condition in which side vision is very blurry or altogether absent.

Injuries and Diseases

The person who has lost one eye must exercise special vigilance to prevent the development of any condition that might affect the sight of the other. Here are a few of the more common conditions to watch out for.

INJURIES. No matter how trivial an injury to your remaining eye may seem to you, have your doctor examine it without delay. Only he can decide whether treatment is needed to ensure the safety of that eye.

Should you ever be so unfortunate as to suffer a major injury to your surviving eye, don't hesitate in authorizing immediate corrective treatment, no matter how hopeless you think your case may be. Saving any vestige of your vision may make the difference in the way you get around for the rest of your life.

INFECTIONS. Any redness of the eye is a signal of *some* trouble. Usually, it's nothing more serious than conjunctivitis, the inflammation of the conjunctiva known as "pink eye." But don't guess at it. Get prompt diagnosis and treatment.

GLAUCOMA. Your ophthalmologist can detect this insidious eye disease long before it does any noticeable damage to your vision — which is one good reason why you should never neglect your regular eye examination. If it's detected early, glaucoma is no cause for the one-eyed patient to despair. Prompt treatment to arrest it, usually by regular use of eyedrops, can prevent it from making any further inroads on your vision for the rest of your life.

CATARACT. This clouding of the lens occurs commonly among older people. When it reaches a point where it interferes significantly with normal visual activity, it can be removed by surgery. This is an operation you can approach with every confidence that your normal vision will be restored with glasses or a contact lens.

DETACHED RETINA. When the retina falls away from its normal position in the eye, it's as if the film were taken out of the camera; vision is lost. But with new techniques using laser beams and freezing instruments, prompt surgery is now remarkably successful in an overwhelming percentage of cases. The patient's normal reading vision and nearly normal side vision can usually be restored.

Other, rarer, eye diseases are equally amenable to treatment or surgery. For all its apparent delicacy, the human eye really is a tough, resilient organ. It heals promptly and completely in most cases. It will work hard for you all through your life, and if you give it — and yourself — reasonable care, you need have no anxiety about its future.

The Royal National Institute for the Blind has worked for years to alert the public about eye hazards, and its advice is of special interest to the one-eyed. The society's recommendations are primarily concerned with wearing safety glasses, observing industrial safety regulations, obeying safety rules pertaining to school shops and laboratories, and paying careful attention to directions for using household cleaning products, aerosol products, insecticides, and herbicides. It particularly cautions against the danger of small objects thrown up by lawn mowers.

The society has made strenuous efforts to assure that children's playthings are safe and to urge strict adult supervision of such activities as playing dart games, air guns, archery and chemistry sets, and missile-type toys. Fireworks, it points out, are responsible for eye injuries to many children each year.

Use of common sense and alertness to potentially hazardous situations will do much to reduce exposure to accidents. It's pleasant to entertain the belief that lightning will not strike the same object twice, but while I was still under medical care as a result of my accident, another bird — this time, a much smaller one — smashed against the windshield of a small aircraft in which I was again riding co-pilot.

The bird struck directly in front of my face. But because of the plane's lower speed, the bird's lighter weight, and the grace of God, its body didn't penetrate the windshield.

14 Seeing to Your Looks

In some cases, the loss of vision on one side has no effect whatever on the appearance and it's practically impossible for any other person to tell which is the "working eye." If you've suffered physical damage, however, or if one eye has been enucleated, or if the area around the eye has been injured, you may have some temporary problems in the way you look.

Modern eye surgery and precision fitting of a prosthesis can virtually eliminate any appearance of imbalance between the two eyes, and plastic surgery can usually repair any damage around the eye socket. So you can nearly always count on regaining a normal appearance in good time.

If the damaged eye remains, there may be some change in appearance caused by the two pupils not tracking precisely in unison. The eyes may seem perfectly aligned when looking straight ahead, but diverge a bit when the good eye glances to one side.

The effect is usually not at all displeasing. In fact, most of us are intrigued by a slight cast in a pleasant face — it seems to add a certain piquancy or individuality. Indeed, Patrick Trevor-Roper, in his book *The World Through Blunted Sight*, notes that earlier societies considered a squint a sign of godliness and beauty. He reminds us that many great artists have gone so far as to portray their subjects with a decided squint that they did not possess in real life.

What makes these observations so important is that the way you look may not be nearly as much of a handicap as the way you *think* you look to others. We all know people who become so uncomfortable under the direct gaze of another person that they'll immediately look away. This natural shyness can be terribly exaggerated for anybody who is unsure of the appearance of his eyes. A determined effort to look people straight in the eye is perhaps the best mental disciple for overcoming this self-consciousness.

"Most important," says Sue Moran, the TV personality mentioned in Chapter 11, "is to look at things and people straight on, turning or raising the whole head and not just the eyes." That's especially important when looking up at someone form, say, a seated position.

Mrs. Moran also has a word of advice to women who may he concerned about the bright look of an artificial eye. "If you're willing to take the time," she says, "you can do a lot with make-up — especially with eye shadow — to make your two eyes look alike. False lashes have also been very useful to me in television and fashion shows — they add shadows and help soften that starry look you sometimes get from a prosthesis."

Sandy Duncan, the TV actress, also makes effective use of false eyelashes. And in a magazine interview, she describes with an inimitable sense of humour the difficulty she has when affixing a strip of eyelashes to the lid of her functioning eye — which must be kept closed during the process.

Television viewers may recall that when she presented Oscars at an Academy Awards ceremony, she wore oversized, tinted glasses. Such glasses were then fashionable. But for Miss Duncan, they also served to soften the glare of the stage lights and to conceal the slight disparity in movement between her two eyes.

Some persons, including Nobel Prize winner Dr. Julius Axelrod, wear glasses with one lens slightly frosted to conceal changes in appearance or movement of a damaged eye. Such a lens is particularly useful if the sightless eye remains sensitive to light.

In our times, the eyepatch seems to be a symbol, not of loss, but of achievement. It endows movie stars and even comic strip characters with an indefinable charisma and is the trademark of famous people who wear it — Moshe Dayan, for example.

For more than 25 years a succession of male models have appeared in innumerable ads wearing a patch over the right eye and looking very distinguished in their sponsor's product, a handsome shirt. The campaign has escalated an obscure Maine shirtmaking company into one of the largest organizations in the business. And one has only to wear an eyepatch himself — and to hear the murmurs of "Ah, the Hathaway Man" — to realize the strength of the identity between symbol and product.

With that campaign, many of the one-eyed suddenly found they possessed a special mystique.

Except in fairly unusual situations, anyone whose eye has been removed can expect to wear an artificial eye. Your ophthalmologist normally will recommend that a prosthetist or artificial eye technician do the fitting. The prescription, selection, and fitting is a matter between these two specialists and they will surely advise you about specific care of the artificial eye and socket. But some background information may be useful.

Surprisingly, the artificial eye is a development of great antiquity, dating back at least to the fifth century B.C. Many materials, including gold, ivory, and porcelain have been used over the centuries, but a type of modern plastic is now considered most satisfactory. Artificial eyes made of plastic can be molded to fit damaged eye sockets better than those made of glass. Glass eyes, too, discolour and roughen after about a year, whereas plastic eyes may last for five years. Furthermore, plastic is less likely to break.

Modern medical science eventually developed techniques for implanting artificial pupils among the muscles so that normal eye movement was restored. These techniques, however, also caused new problems, particularly in maintaining proper hygiene. So the design of conventional artificial eyes has been improved to provide a satisfactory degree of eye movement. As pointed out earlier in this chapter, such movement can be greatly aided by turning or raising the head toward the subject being viewed rather than turning just the eyes.

In selecting a matching eye, it's important to rely on the advice of your prosthetist or artificial eye technician. If he recommends an eye with a pupil slightly smaller than your natural eye, it's because experience has taught him that it will reduce the tendency toward an appearance of a "stare" and so attract less attention. He may be looking for a pleasing effect rather than an exact match. So trust his skill and judgment and you'll find that it will pay dividends in improved appearance.

Most artificial eyes are worn continuously, day and night, and are removed only for cleaning. Your ophthalmologist will advise you on your specific case.

When wiping your artificial eye, remember to always wipe *toward* the nose. Otherwise you may dislodge the eye and cause it to rotate to an incorrect position with rather bizarre results.

15 Driver and Pilot Licensing Standards

"Will I be able to drive?"

That is one of the first questions likely to be asked by the person who has lost the use of one eye.

The short answer is PROBABLY.

The current regulations allow that provided that the sight in the remaining eye meets the acuity standards of the Driver Vehicle Licencing Agency (DVLA) there are no restrictions on a person's licence. This applies to PCV and HGV categories as well. The present requirement is the capability to read a car number plate from 20.5 metres.

The wise driver should, at his own expense, to have an optical examination done by his physician or optometrist to determine that the driver's vision meets the standard.

Should the driver pass the test, then no further action is required. However, if the driver does not meet the standard, then the DVLA must be advised and a copy of the optical examination report sent to:

Driver Vehicle Licencing Agency
Longview Road
Morriston
Swansea, Wales
SA6 7JL

You are required to notify your insurance company to ensure that your coverage is maintained. This can be done through your agent. Make sure you do this as it could be devastating to be in an accident and find your insurance does not cover you because you did not notify them of the change in your status.

The American Association of Motor Vehicle Administrators and the American Optometric Association, in a jointly published booklet on visual screening for driver licensing, remark that "most drivers are anxious to retain driving privileges and as a result they learn to compensate for deficiencies."

Referring specifically to the one-eyed driver, the booklet states: "Since there is greatly impaired space perception, the person usually learns to utilize other cues such as shadows and perspective. One-eyed drivers learn or should be instructed to turn their head from side to side frequently, especially if the left eye is the blind one. The reason for this seems to be that there may be more unobserved hazards approaching form the left side. A further safeguard for the one-eyed driver is the use of outside rearview mirrors."

Most new cars now come equipped with a left-hand mirror which is remote controlled. If your new car is not factory equipped with this aid, you can have your dealer install one for you. For any older model that does not have a second mirror, you can find a suitable unit at most shops selling car accessories or at your dealer.

Meanwhile, when driving cars other than my own, I use a small, lightweight clamp-on mirror that I bought in a local spare parts shop.

There are some wide angle mirrors on the market that fit over the standard rear view mirror. They provide a door to door view of what is on both sides of you as well as what is behind you. These mirrors when used in conjunction with your two adjustable side mirrors provide almost a 180 degree field of vision.

The Highway Research Board Bulletin describes the experience of a researcher who, a few years ago, conducted driving experiments with one eye covered. He concluded that a wide-angle rear view mirror located so that it can be used without the driver shifting his head was helpful. He also found that a conventional mirror with individually adjustable side wings is of definite value.

If you have to have an outside left-side mirror, you can better take advantage of its limited usefulness if you have it installed far enough forward — within your horizontal field — so you can see it without turning your head. Simply note what's the limit of your vision of the left when you're looking straight ahead, and have the mirror placed a little ahead of that point.

One side benefit of an outside mirror on the left is that you can use its protrusion to check your clearance of that side when you're pulling up next to a wall or alongside a parked car.

Pilot Licensing Standards

The International Civil Aviation Organization is the agency of the United Nations responsible for adopting standards and recommended practices for safe, efficient, regular and economic international civil aviation operation.

The ICAO visual regulations require vision in both eyes. Therefore, monocular pilots are considered as not meeting minimum international standards for commercial pilots. However participating nations have the prerogative to allow exemptions based on medical dispensation to allow monocular pilots. These licenses would be recognized by the ICAO as valid.

The United Kingdom, one of several nations that takes an enlightened attitude about one-eyed fliers, has certified one-eyed persons not only as private fliers but also as commercial and air transport rated pilots. Monocular persons may be certified as private pilots and for night instrument rating. However, a monocular person would have an application for a professional pilot's licence refused.

All pilots in the United Kingdom are required to advise the licensing authority immediately upon accident or injury or after sickness absence in excess of twenty consecutive days.

In the case of a licensed pilot losing the sight of one eye, an ophthalmic examination is necessary before the licence may be reissued. A private pilot may have this examination done by a local consultant. Professional aircrew would have this examination done by the ophthalmologist at the national centre of the Civil Aviation Authority. A period of six months is required to allow the pilot to adjust to monocular vision before retesting. A medical flight test will be necessary to demonstrate adaptability to flying with monocular vision.

There will also be some restrictions placed on the licence of a monocular pilot.

"While flying in United Kingdom airspace the monocular private pilot is required to wear thin framed protective spectacles and must have protective goggles available at all times. The goggles must be worn during any contingency involving risk to eyesight, including negative or zero G manoeuvres."

Professional pilots would be restricted to "flying as or with a qualified co-pilot"

For more detailed information I suggest you contact:

Civil Aviation Authority
Aviation House
South Area
Gatwick Airport
West Sussex RH6 0YR

Phone (0293) 567171
Fax (0293) 573999
Telex 878753

In a carefully controlled experiment, pilots with normal vision were asked to make a series of landings. After their performances were meticulously evaluated and recorded, they were told to repeat the landings with one eye covered. Their performance scores were identical, even though the pilots complained that the one-eye landings were more difficult. That's hardly surprising, considering that they were completely unadapted to monocular vision.

Those tests used experienced NASA research pilots as subjects, and it was speculated that their skill influenced the results. Accordingly, additional, carefully controlled tests were conducted, and an *Aerospace Medicine* report describes them: Thirty pilots — 27 men and three women — were selected because of their limited flying experience; none had more than 500 hours total flying time, about half had less than 100 hours. The tests included six landings for each subject with normal vision, six landings with the right eye covered, and six landings with the left eye covered. The pilots were to try to touch down as accurately as possible on a designated spot on the runway.

The astonishing conclusion, reached with a high degree of statistical certainty, was that landing performance is *not* degraded by the transition from binocular to monocular vision; *in fact, under the conditions of this test, performance actually improved.*

The research team further concluded that:

• Flying experience doesn't have any effect on monocular performance.

• Eye dominance doesn't affect monocular landing performance.

• Linear perspective is the dominant visual mechanism to provide distance cues during landing.

Although there were too few women in the tests to provide statistical significance, their performance far surpassed that of the male average.

It's likely that when they had one eye covered the participants were trying hard, probably much harder than usual, to do a good job. The message here is that with extra effort and concentration, even very difficult tasks can be executed.

Today the Civil Aviation Authority does not withhold licences because of monocular vision. However, there have been cases where an unfavourable finding by an eye specialist has resulted in the refusal to issue or renew a monocular pilot's licence.

Glider pilots and balloonists also need licences.

Recently, in Canada, I took my family hot-air ballooning. During the traditional champagne picnic (held to celebrate a successful flight and landing), I discovered that our pilot, John Medlock, is known as "The World's Only One-eyed Tasmanian Professional Hot-Air Balloon Pilot". This charming young Australian lost the sight in his right eye, as a child, due to an accident. He earned his private pilot licence in Australia, then went to England, where he managed a pub until he acquired his hot air balloon pilot licence.

John works around the world piloting hot-air balloons. He is a great example of what can be accomplished in spite of what is often perceived as a handicap.

16 For Parents Only

What can parents tell a child who has just lost and eye? If they haven't had — and, of course, this is usually the case — the same experience, it's hard for them to talk about it. In any case, they should approach the subject with care and sensitivity, since damage to the child's emotional outlook can be greater than the physical loss of the eye and last just as long.

To get a better understanding of the problem, I talked with parents, pediatric ophthalmologists, psychiatrists, people who as children had lost an eye, and — perhaps most revealing of all — youngsters who had just lost an eye. There seems to be general agreement on several points: Discussions of the loss must be adjusted according to the child's age, sex, emotional stability, maturity, natural co-ordination, athletic inclination, and the child-parent relationship. Moreover, if parents recognize the true impact of the eye loss, this will help them maintain a calm, dispassionate attitude that can prevent the build-up of exaggerated fears. Certainly, emotional displays in the presence of the child are out of order. They all agree that children, in general, adapt quickly, and that the younger the child, the quicker and more complete is the adaptation.

Parents who tend to be overprotective can learn a few things from the example of Congressman Morris Udall, a 1976 candidate for his party's Presidential nomination. When I met with him in his Capitol Hill office, he recounted his own experience. His right eye was severely injured in an accident when he was six, and he finally lost it after some harrowing treatment. In successful support of the court case of a one-eyed athlete who had been barred from a university basketball team because of the institution's protectionist policy, Congressman Udall wrote the following account of his own success in sports.

Statement by Congressman Morris K. Udall
Member of Congress
Second District of Arizona

At the age of six, I suffered a serious injury to my right eye which eventually led to surgery to remove the eye. The loss of the eye, however, never interfered with my ability or opportunity to engage in athletic events in high school, college, or as a professional. I can also state unequivocally that the wearing of a glass eye never led to or contributed to any injury in athletic competition.

In high school, in St. John's, Arizona, I played quarterback on the football team and was also captain of the basketball team. While at the University of Arizona, I played three years of university basketball and even led the team in scoring one of those years. In fact, my shooting proficiency on the basketball court was good enough to bring an allegation by a rival fan that "Udall can't shoot that well with only one eye."

Although my college career was interrupted by service in the Army Air Corps during World War II, I continued to play basketball while in the Army and organized a team at Fort Huachuca, Arizona, which was, in part, made up of one-eyed players.

After college, I played a year of professional basketball in 1948-49 with the then Denver Nuggets of the National Basketball League.

In addition, I obtained a private pilot's license in 1946, which I still hold, and have logged more than 4,000 hours of flight time.

While my career has been in law and public service, in my opinion the loss of an eye did not and would not have interfered with my ability to compete professionally in athletics, nor did it lead to any injuries.

Acting on behalf of the one-eyed college basketball player is typical of Mo Udall. Whenever parents ask, he writes to encourage kids who've lost vision in one eye.

Udall credits his mother with "doing all the right things" following the accident. He said that she never restricted his activities. She allowed his to play normally and, as he grew older, to engage in sports. When I asked Udall if his drive to overcome his disadvantage played a role in his achievements, he said he was determined as a youngster to show that he could do anything anybody else could do, and probably better. He now believes that his drive to compensate pushed him farther than he otherwise would have gone.

I've had occasion to appear as an expert witness in eye-loss court cases. I recognize the need for just compensation and I know that litigation can't in every case be avoided, but I believe every effort should be made to spare a child from direct involvement in court proceedings. Parents must weigh the risk of damage to a child's psyche against prospects for a settlement and not hesitate to forgo litigation if the risk is too great.

A final point: Children can cruelly tease one of their number about a physical characteristic that sets him apart from the crowd. A one-eyed child is likely to be the subject of such attacks, particularly if his condition is made obvious by bandages, special glasses, and the like. Since it's impractical and undesirable to isolate the child, a little advance home coaching can help. If he's got self-confidence, our one-eyed victim of teasing can laugh it off. Make sure the child realizes that monocularity sets few limitations and is quite common among people in all walks of life. Let him know, too, that he's in great company.

17 Great Company

Throughout history people with all kinds of handicaps have distinguished themselves in all walks of life, and in this book I've cited the accomplishments of just some public figures, entertainers, scientists, pilots, and athletes who have overcome the problem and inconvenience of one-eyed sight. For the person who has just joined this club, it may be interesting and encouraging to note a few of its more prominent members and the diversity of their accomplishments. I don't say that losing an eye can make you great, but if you want to make your mark, the loss needn't stop you.

Archibald Percival Wavell, soldier, administrator, poet and former viceroy of India.

Herbert Morrison, British Labour Party statesman, foreign secretary, deputy prime minister.

Joe Davis, World snooker champion and holder of

the record for highest score on break.

Rex Harrison, distinguished stage and screen actor probably best remembered for his role as Professor Henry Higgins in "My Fair Lady".

Eric J. Hoskins, International bird photographer and ornithologist, recognized for his pioneering work in developing new techniques for flash lighting and cinematography of birds.

Theodore Roosevelt, the vigorous U.S. President who, while in office, lost his left eye in a boxing bout with a naval officer.

Moshe Dayan, Israeli military leader and statesman. A World War II gunfire accident took his left eye but didn't dampen a distinguished public career.

Ian Smith, prime minister of Rhodesia, centre of worldwide controversy.

Morris K. Udall, congressman and 1976 candidate for Presidential nomination, who lost his right eye at age six, but didn't let that keep him from scholastic and professional athletics, flying, and public service.

Sammy Davis Jr., the irrepressible entertainer who didn't achieve superstardom until after an automobile accident cost him the sight of his left eye.

John Ford, top movie director.

Peter Falk, plodding star of the long-running TV series "Columbo," who solves crimes with one eye.

Hilaire Germain Edgar Degas, master French impressionist who did some of his finest work after he lost his right eye in the siege of Paris.

John Milton, 17th-century poet.

Julius Axelrod, 1970 Nobel Prize winner in physiology and medicine, whose graduate work and Nobel Prize efforts came after a laboratory accident in which he lost his left eye.

Guglielmo Marconi, inventor of the radio.

Wiley Post, pioneering aviator who, with vision only in his right eye, made the first solo circumnavigation of the globe in seven days, 18 hours, 49 minutes. Post made many contributions to flight technology.

Horatio Nelson, the greatest of British naval heroes, whose victory at Trafalgar occurred more than 10 years after he lost his right eye in battle off Corsica.

Nelson even used his blind eye to advantage in the historic Battle of Copenhagen in 1801. His superior, Sir Hyde Parker, had signalled him to halt his attack on a Danish ship against what Parker considered very dubious odds. Nelson placed a telescope against his blind eye, and after a careful "look," told his aide, "I do not see the signal." He then proceeded with the attack, which was soon to become a major chapter in Britain's proud naval history.

Thus Nelson used his handicap to turn a potential defeat into a resounding victory.

Go, and do thou likewise.